The Pediatric Nursing Skills Manual

The Pediatric Nursing Skills Manual

BETTY JO WHITSON, R.N., M.N.
Clinical Specialist—Pediatric Nursing
Associate Professor of Pediatric Nursing
Chairman, Division of Nursing
University of South Carolina at Aiken

JUDITH M. MCFARLANE, R.N., M.N.
Doctoral Candidate, School of Public Health
The University of Texas Health Science Center at
 Houston
Formerly Assistant Professor and Pediatric
 Clinical Specialist in Hematology
Medical College of Georgia, Augusta, Georgia

A WILEY MEDICAL PUBLICATION
JOHN WILEY & SONS
New York · Chichester · Brisbane · Toronto

Library of Congress Cataloging in Publication Data

Whitson, Betty Jo.
   The pediatric nursing skills manual.

   (A Wiley medical publication)
   Includes index.
   1.   Pediatric nursing—Handbooks, manuals, etc.
I.   McFarlane, Judith, joint author.   II.   Title.
[DNLM: 1.   Pediatric nursing.   WY159 W623p]
RJ245.W48   610.73′62   79-27079
ISBN 0-471-04511-X

Printed in the United States of America

10 9 8 7 6 5 4 3 2 1

For my husband, Warren, for loving, encouraging, and enduring; for Robert, John, and Jim; and of course, for "Butch"

BJW

For my children, Scott and Heather

JMMcF

Preface

Pediatric nursing presents a special challenge in that many nursing procedures and techniques that are suitable for adult nursing are simply not appropriate to the nursing of children, for example, the administration of medications, the application of restraints, and feeding techniques.

The primary objective of this manual is to give the nursing student, as well as the practicing nurse, a practical and easy-to-use guide to those procedures that are unique to pediatric nursing.

This comprehensive guide was conceived as a companion to *Contemporary Pediatric Nursing: A Conceptual Approach*, by Judith McFarlane, Betty Jo Whitson, and Lucy M. Hartley (John Wiley, 1980), although it can be used in conjunction with any other pediatric nursing text or by itself. This volume is selective in that it makes no attempt to include nursing procedures normally discussed in adult nursing procedure manuals, nor does it cover such specialized skills as neonatal intensive care or physical assessment.

Since procedures and equipment vary with institutions, some of the techniques described herein must be used as guidelines; the reader, of necessity, will adapt some instructions in this manual to suit the procedures and brands of equipment used in her institution.

Over 200 illustrations, most of them prepared especially for this manual, accompany brief, straightforward explanations of the skills discussed here. In many cases, several steps of the procedure are illustrated. We are confident that this format will provide the reader with an optimal guide to the essential skills of pediatric nursing.

B.J.W.
J.M.McF.

Acknowledgments

We wish to thank the following people for their help and support in the completion of this book: The Wiley staff, especially Cathy Somer for initiating the project, Don Schott for editing the manuscript and Eileen Tommaso for piloting the text through production. For reviewing the manuscript: Lucy M. Hartley, R.N., M.N., Assistant Professor, University of South Carolina, College of Nursing, and Family Nurse Specialist, 7 Oaks Family Practice Center, Columbia, S.C.; Van Inglett, R.N., B.S.N., Director of Pediatric Nursing, University Hospital, Augusta, Georgia; Linda M. Fleming, R.N., M.S.N., Supervisor, Obstetrical Nursing, St. Anthony Hospital, Denver, Colorado; Vickie Amerson, R.N., B.S.N., Nursing Manager, Pediatric-Adolescent Unit, University Hospital, Augusta, Georgia; Barbara McAdams, R.N., Nursing Manager, Pediatric Unit, University Hospital, Augusta, Georgia; Nell Adams, R.N., Nursing Manager, Pediatric Intensive Care Unit, University Hospital, Augusta, Georgia; Francis Bowers, R.N., Day Shift Supervisor, Pediatric-Adolescent Unit, University

Hospital, Augusta, Georgia; and Josephine Phillips, R.N.

Medical illustrators from the Division of Health Communications, Medical College of Georgia, Augusta, Georgia: David Mascaro, John Hagen, Leslie Dessauer, and Karen Waldo.

Typists: Karen Harley and Donna Weatherford.

We also wish to thank our students for their enthusiasm and support; our families and friends for encouraging, loving, and doing without during the preparation of this book; and a special thanks to our patients and teachers—the children with whom we have worked, laughed, and cried over the years.

B.J.W.
J.M.McF.

Contents

CHAPTER 1

Observation of the Child

VITAL SIGNS

Temperature

The child, especially the preschooler, views temperature taking as an intrusive procedure and may even resist axillary temperature measurements.

The young infant may have little or no fever even with severe infections, while the older infant and the child tend to have much higher temperatures than adults. The older infant and child may have a high fever during a benign illness too.

In most cases, the infant's and young child's temperature is measured rectally. However, rectal measurement is contraindicated if the child has diarrhea, has had recent rectal surgery, has rectal ulcers (as in leukemia), or weighs less than 1.8 kg (4 pounds). Remember that readings may be altered by the presence of feces. Care must be taken not to damage the rectal mucosa. The normal range for temperature measured rectally is 36.2° to 37.8° C (97° to 100° F). (See Table 1-1 for Celsius and Fahrenheit equivalents.)

Table 1-1 Equivalent Temperature Readings

Celsius [a] (°C)		Fahrenheit [a] (°F)	
0	32.0	39.0	102.2
20.	68.0	39.2	102.6
30.	86.0	39.4	103.
31.	87.8	39.6	103.3
32.	89.6	39.8	103.7
33.	91.4	40.0	104.
34.	93.2	40.2	104.4
35.	95.0	40.4	104.7
36.	96.8	40.5	105.0
37.	98.6	40.6	105.1
37.2	99.	40.8	105.4
37.4	99.3	41.0	105.8
37.6	99.7	41.2	106.2
37.7	100.0	41.4	106.5
37.8	100.1	41.6	106.9
38.0	100.4	41.8	107.2
38.2	100.8	42.	107.6
38.4	101.2	43.	109.4
38.6	101.5	44.	111.2
38.8	102.	100.	212.

[a]To convert Celsius readings to Fahrenheit, multiply by 1.8 and add 32. To convert Fahrenheit readings to Celsius, subtract 32 and divide by 1.8.

Axillary temperature measurements are taken routinely in premature and neonatal nurseries. There is no danger of perforating the rectum or colon, but obtaining an accurate reading takes longer than does a rectal reading. The normal range for axillary readings is 35.9° to 36.7° C (96.6° to 98.0° F).

Temperature is measured orally if the child is old enough to refrain from biting the thermometer and can cooperate by keeping the thermometer under his tongue and keeping his lips closed. Although an oral reading more closely approximates arterial temperature, it is readily influenced by the ingestion of hot or cold fluids, by oxygen therapy, or by the presence of a nasogastric tube. Use another method if the child has difficulty breathing, if he has had oral surgery, or if he is receiving oxygen. The normal range for oral readings is 36.4° to 37.4° C (97.6° to 99.3° F).

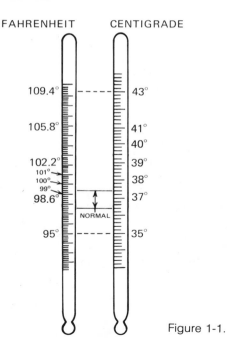

Figure 1-1.

Glass Thermometer
Conventional glass thermometers (Figure 1-1) measure temperature on the Celsius and Fahrenheit scales.

Procedure to Measure Rectal Temperature

1. With the child supine, hold the legs firmly around the ankles with one hand (Figure 1-2). With the child in this position (rather than prone), you can talk to or otherwise interact with him during the procedure.
2. With the other hand, gently insert just the bulb of the lubricated thermometer into the anus about ¼ to ½ inch. (Lubrication with a water-soluble jelly is preferred.)

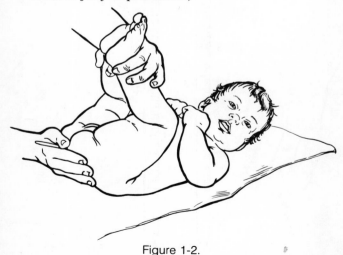

Figure 1-2.

3. Hold the thermometer securely in place for three to five minutes, gently pressing the buttocks together with the heel of hand and fingers; this pressure helps prevent the child from defecating or pushing the thermometer out during the procedure.

4. Read temperature and wipe thermometer clean.

5. Clothe the child.

6. Wash hands and record temperature as follows:
   37.8°C ®

Procedure to Measure Axillary Temperature

1. Place bulb of thermometer on the child's unwashed axilla (Figure 1-3). (Washing before pro-

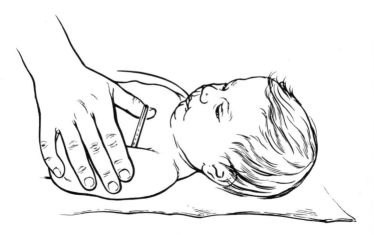

Figure 1-3.

cedure may result in a false low reading.) Hold the child's arm firmly against his side to secure thermometer. Keep in place 9 to 11 minutes.

2. Read and record temperature as follows:
   36.7°C⒜

Procedure to Measure Oral Temperature

Proceed as you would with an adult, placing thermometer under the right side of the tongue (close to the sublingual artery). Remind the child to keep the thermometer under his tongue, not to bite the thermometer, and to keep his lips closed. Leave the thermometer in place for five minutes.

Uni-Temp Thermometer

The Uni-Temp thermometer (Figure 1-4) is a flat, plastic and aluminum single-use thermometer. The aluminum is treated with chemicals that make it sensitive to temperature. The Uni-Temp is accurate to within 0.2°F and registers oral temperatures in

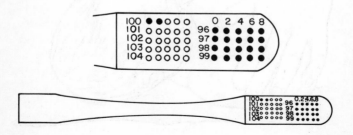

Figure 1-4.

one minute and axillary temperatures in three minutes. The Uni-Temp cannot be used rectally.

Because of its safety, shape, and the speed with which it registers temperature, the Uni-Temp is particularly suited for use with children. Fahrenheit and Celsius models are available.

Procedure for Using Uni-Temp Thermometer

Place dotted end of Uni-Temp thermometer at base of tongue for one full minute or flat in axilla for three minutes.

The Uni-Temp thermometer has a series of yellow dots corresponding to temperatures from 96.0° to 104.8°F. The dots turn red as they register heat. Six seconds after removal from the patient's mouth or axilla, the dots stabilize, leaving both red and yellow dots. The red dot with the highest value indicates the patient's temperature. The thermometer shown in Figure 1-4 registers 100.2°F.

IVAC Electronic Clinical Thermometer

The IVAC Electronic Clinical Thermometer is a self-contained unit with a rechargeable battery. Both Celsius and Fahrenheit units are available. The unit comes with blue oral probes and red rectal probes that are used with disposable probe covers. An audible tone signals that the temperature has been computed; the temperature appears on the digital display screen. (Figures 1-5, 1-6, 1-7, 1-8, 1-9, and 1-10, and the following instructions for the use of the IVAC Electronic Clinical Thermometer are reproduced by permission of IVAC Corporation.)

Procedure for Using IVAC Electronic Clinical Thermometer

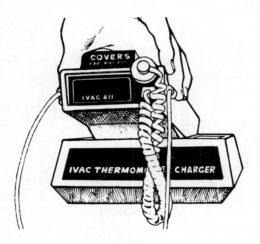

Figure 1-5.

Remove thermometer from charger and place carrying strap around your neck (Figure 1-5).

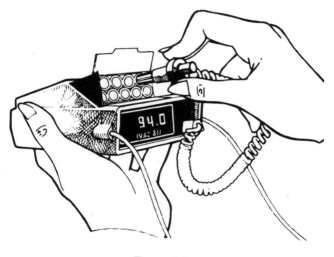

Figure 1-6.

Grasp probe by large ring at top. Attach a disposable probe cover by inserting probe firmly into probe cover (Figure 1-6). Do not push top—it is the ejection button.

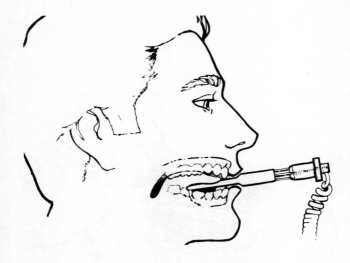

Figure 1-7.

For oral temperatures, slowly slide probe under the front of the child's tongue and along the gum line to the sublingual pocket at base of tongue (Figure 1-7). The child's lips should come to rest at the step on the probe cover. For rectal temperatures, follow similar technique, except use red colored probe. Use current techniques for penetration.

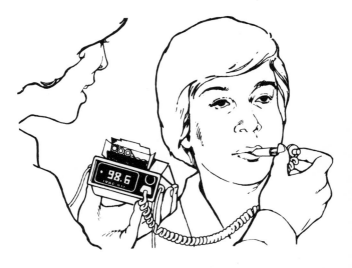

Figure 1-8.

Hold the probe! Do not watch digital display panel; maintain position of probe in the patient until audible signal notifies you that child's temperature has been reached and is displayed (Figure 1-8).

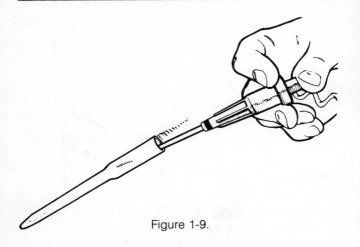

Figure 1-9.

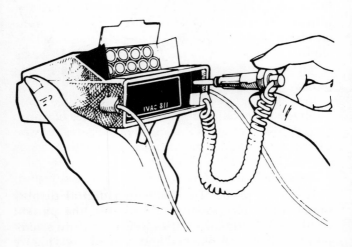

Figure 1-10.

Remove probe from the child's mouth. Discard probe cover by pushing ejection button with thumb (Figure 1-9).

After reading and recording temperature, return probe to its storage well. This will automatically turn thermometer off (Figure 1-10). After completing temperature rounds, return thermometer to charging base.

Pulse

Pulse rate, rhythm, and quality are recorded routinely. The force and quality are usually more significant in the young child than is the rate. A slight irregularity during sleep is not significant, but a slow, constantly irregular pulse is always significant. Pulse rate varies with respiration in most children, and it tends to be greatly increased by slight disturbances; it may rise by 20 to 30 beats when the child is approached by a stranger (or his nurse).

In addition, pulse rates increase by 8 to 10 beats a minute for each degree of fever. In cases of upper airway obstruction in the child, pulse rates may be 140 to 160; with lower airway obstruction, rates may be 180 to 200 or higher.

Take the apical pulse in infants for one full minute. Unless the older child has problems with oxygenation, his pulse may be counted for 30 seconds and multiplied by two. (See Table 1-2 for average pulse rates at rest.) Always take the pulse before the temperature to obtain the most accurate measurement. Recall that temperature taking is intrusive and will upset the child, resulting in an elevated pulse.

Table 1-2 **Average Pulse Rates at Rest**

Age	Range	Average
Newborn	70-170	120
1-11 months	80-160	120
2 years	80-130	110
4 years	80-120	100
6 years	75-115	100
8-10 years	70-110	90
12 years[a]	70-110	90
14 years	65-105	85
16 years	60-100	80
18 years	55-95	75

[a]From age 12 to 18 years, boys' rates are five points lower.

Procedure for Pulse Taking

Palpate the child's left chest wall to determine the point of maximum impulse (PMI), where you can best feel the heartbeat. Place diaphragm of stethoscope on the chest over the PMI and count the pulse for one minute (Figure 1-11).

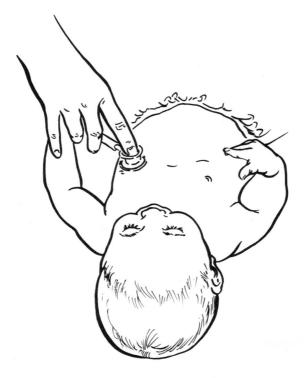

Figure 1-11.

If diaphragm of stethoscope is too large for the child's chest, it will not form a seal, and heart sounds will be heard with difficulty or not at all (Figure 1-12).

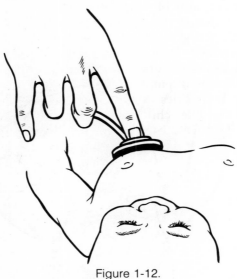

Figure 1-12.

Respirations

The rate, depth, rhythm, and quality of respirations are routinely noted. Rates in infants are higher than in adults, and the rhythm is irregular, especially in the premature or very young infant. Until the age of seven, respiratory movement is abdominal; after age seven, movement is primarily costal. The respiration-to-pulse ratio is normally 1:4. Each degree of fever increases the respiratory rate by four breaths/min. The rate of respiration varies from 30 to 50 breaths/min at birth, 16 to 20 at six years of age, and 14 to 16 at puberty.

Do not disturb the child when observing his respirations, since respirations will increase if the child is upset or excited. Count respirations for one full minute for the infant; for the older child, count for 30 seconds and multiply the result by two. Note whether both sides of the chest move symmetrically. If the older child uses abdominal breathing, suspect dyspnea. Listen for respiratory noises such as wheezing, stridor, or grunting. Observe for signs of dyspnea (restlessness, retractions, nasal flaring, and cyanosis).

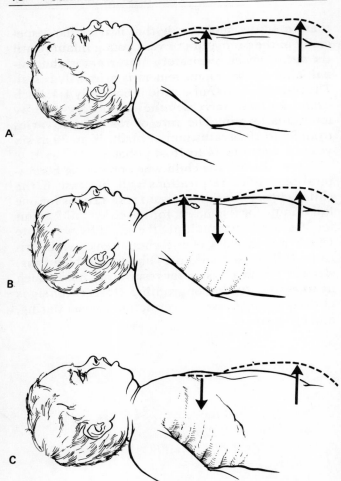

Figure 1-13.

Figures 1-13, 1-14, and 1-15 illustrate the criteria used to evaluate respiratory distress. The scoring system shown below will yield a score between zero and 10. On each criterion, a score of zero indicates no difficulty; a score of 1 indicates moderate difficulty; and a score of 2 indicates maximum difficulty. Scores are given for the following criteria: upper chest movement, lower chest retractions, xiphoid retractions, expiratory grunt, and flaring nares. A total score of zero indicates no distress; a total score of 10 indicates maximum respiratory distress.

◀ Figure 1-13

a:	Synchronized movement of upper chest and abdomen	0
	No lower chest retractions	0
b:	Lag on inspiration	1
	Lower chest retractions just visible	1
c:	Seesaw movement of chest and abdomen	2
	Marked lower chest retractions	2

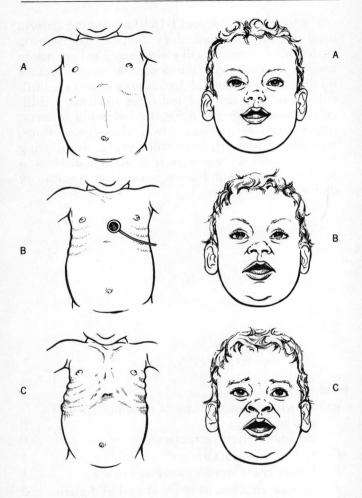

Figure 1-14.   Figure 1-15.

Figure 1-14

a:	No xiphoid retractions	0
	No expiratory grunt	0
b:	Xiphoid retractions just visible	1
	Expiratory grunt audible with stethoscope	1
c:	Marked xiphoid and sternal retractions	2
	Expiratory grunt audible with unaided ear	2

Figure 1-15

a:	No flaring of nares	0
b:	Minimal flaring of nares	1
c:	Marked flaring of nares	2

Blood Pressure

Procedures different from those used in adults are necessary for the reliable measurement of blood pressure in children and adolescents. Characteristics in children that can affect blood pressure readings are their size, anxiety in unfamiliar situations, and the difficulty of hearing Korotkoff sounds (heart phases I, IV, and V). Systolic pressure (phase I) is measured when the first consecutive sounds are heard. Korotkoff sound IV is the muffled sound; Korotkoff sound V is the disappearance of sound. Because heart sounds are often heard throughout deflation, the Korotkoff sound IV is used for the diastolic reading in children. If all three sounds are audible, record them as 116/76/56 (I/IV/V). Figures 1-16 and 1-17 show percentiles of blood pressure in females and males.

Equipment

Cuff
Stethoscope
Sphygmomanometer
Ultrasound unit
Elastic bandage

The width of the cuff should cover two thirds of the upper arm or leg and should be at least 20 percent longer than the limb's diameter. A cuff that is too large will result in minimal error, but a cuff that is too small will result in erroneously high readings. Leave 1 centimeter in the antecubital or popliteal fossa for proper placement of the stetho-

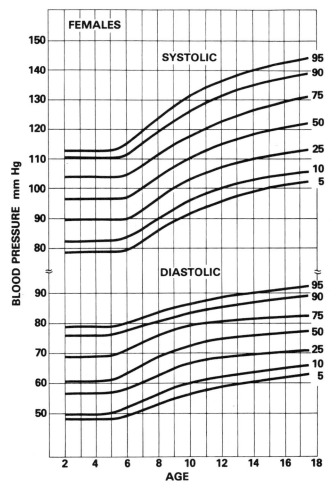

Figure 1-16. Percentiles of blood pressure measurement (right arm, seated). (The National Heart, Lung, and Blood Institute's Task Force on Blood Pressure Control in Children: Report of the Task Force on Blood Pressure Control in Children, *Pediatrics* 59(Suppl):797–820, 1977.)

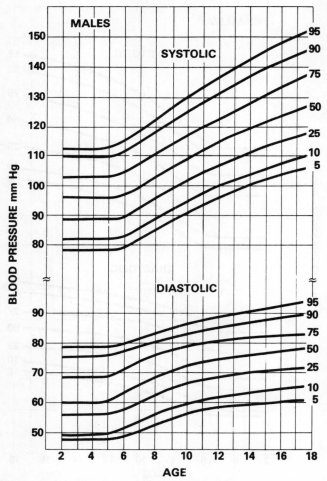

Figure 1-17. Percentiles of blood pressure measurement (right arm, seated). (The National Heart, Lung, and Blood Institute's Task Force on Blood Pressure Control in Children: Report of the Task Force on Blood Pressure Control in Children, *Pediatrics* 59(Suppl):797–820, 1977.)

scope. Size of the arm or leg, rather than age of the child, is the determining factor.

The range of cuff sizes is:

Cuff Name	Width (cm)	Length (cm)
Newborn	2.5– 4.0	5.0–10.0
Infant	6.0– 8.0	12.0–13.5
Child	9.0–10.0	17.0–22.5

Procedure for Flush Method

This method is used for infants less than one year of age when ultrasound equipment is not available. Flush pressure approximates the mean arterial pressure. It is usually less than 80 mmHg in infants under one year of age.

Place proper-size cuff on the infant's upper arm or forearm (Figure 1-18).

Elevate the arm and, beginning at the hand, wrap an elastic bandage tightly around the hand

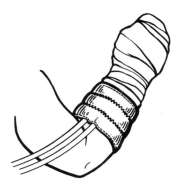

Figure 1-18.

and forearm to force the blood into the upper arm. The hand and forearm will pale.

Rapidly inflate the cuff and remove the bandage (Figure 1-19).

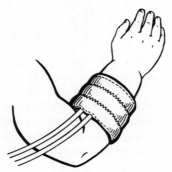

Figure 1-19.

Slowly deflate the cuff. Record flush pressure when hand and forearm flush (become pink) (Figure 1-20).

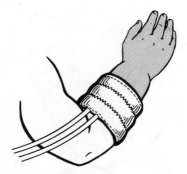

Figure 1-20.

Procedure for Auscultation

For the child three years of age and older, this is the preferred method. Let the child sit during the procedure, rather than lie down, giving him more control over his environment. Give the child time to become familiar with the equipment and to relax. Reassure him that the procedure is painless.

Wrap the proper-size cuff around the right arm and hold the arm level with the heart. Palpate the brachial artery with one hand and rapidly inflate and deflate the cuff to obtain a rough estimate of the systolic pressure. Place the stethoscope over the artery and inflate the cuff to just a few mmHg above estimated systolic pressure. Deflate at 2 mmHg/sec. Blood pressure is charted as follows:

Sitting position: right arm: 9-cm cuff:
116/76/56 (I/IV/V)

Procedure for Palpation

If blood pressure cannot be auscultated, palpate the mean arterial pressure. Place the cuff on the child's arm, palpate the brachial artery, and inflate the cuff. The pressure is read when the pulse returns to the artery during deflation of the cuff.

Procedure for Thigh Measurement

Blood pressure may be measured in the thigh with
the stethoscope over the femoral artery in the popliteal space (Figure 1-21). Pressure will be the same
as that derived from arm readings if the infant is
less than one year of age. After one year, systolic
pressure in the leg will be about 20 mmHg higher,
while diastolic pressure will be the same as that in
the arm.

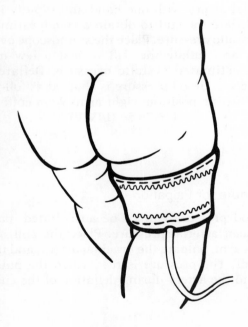

Figure 1-21.

Procedure for Ultrasound Measurement

Ultrasound is a reliable method for measuring blood pressure, especially in premature and full-term infants. However, some equipment measures only systolic pressure.

With the arteriosonde Model 1020 Blood Pressure Monitor, a portable blood pressure unit by Roche Medical Electronics, Inc. (Figure 1-22), ultrasonically detected arterial wall motion is converted to digital displays on a screen. Both systolic and diastolic pressures are recorded. Cuff sizes include premature arm, neonatal arm/premature thigh, infant arm/neonatal thigh, pediatric arm/infant thigh, and several adult sizes. Transducers (Figure 1-23) are available in three sizes: neonatal (A) (for limb circumferences of less than 9 cm); infant (B) (for limb circumferences of 9 to 16 centimeters); and pediatric/adult (C). Neonatal and infant transducers snap onto the cuff (D), and the pediatric/adult transducer attaches with Velcro.

1. Obtain proper-size cuff and transducer.
2. Attach transducer to cuff (E), being sure transducer is free of gel residue.
3. Apply thin, continuous layer of Gelisonde Ultrasonic Coupling Gel to face of transducer (F).
4. Palpate desired artery and place transducer over artery. (For remainder of this procedure, refer to Figure 1-22.) Wrap cuff (A) snugly around limb, being careful not to move transducer.

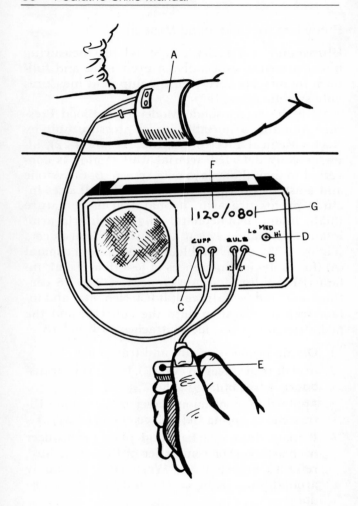

Figure 1-22.

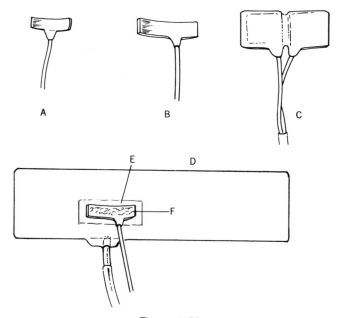

A   B   C

E   D

F

Figure 1-23.

5. Attach hand bulb assembly to BULB connections (B).
6. Attach cuff assembly to CUFF connections (C).
7. Set sensitivity switch (D) at MED for normal infants and children and at HI for prematures, neonates, and weak infants.
8. Plug machine into a three-prong power receptacle, or operate on battery power, provided battery meter registers in green zone.

9. Hold limb still during procedure to avoid distortion of sound.

10. Inflate cuff to 30 mmHg above anticipated systolic pressure.

11. Bleed off pressure at 2 to 3 mmHg/sec. When first sounds are heard, depress "display lock" button (E) to lock systolic digits (F) at systolic pressure. Diastolic digits will then light and begin to bleed off.

12. When phase IV sounds (muffling) are heard, depress "display lock" button again to lock diastolic digits (G) at diastolic pressure.

13. Record pressure readings, then dump remaining cuff pressure. Instrument will turn off when pressure is dumped.

14. Remove cuff assembly and clean transducer with damp cloth.

15. Wipe child's arm to remove gel residue.

NURSING MEASURES FOR ELEVATED TEMPERATURES

If the child has a fever, check his temperature every hour (using the same method each time) until it is stable, then every two hours until it returns to normal, then every four hours for 24 hours. If the child appears uncomfortable or toxic, initiate measures to reduce the fever.

1. Offer clear fluids to prevent dehydration.

2. Dress the child in lightweight clothes to expose skin to air, thereby increasing heat loss.

3. Give a sponge bath if ordered (procedure follows) to lower temperature by promoting evaporation of water from the skin.

4. Give antipyretic drugs as ordered.

5. Use a hypothermia blanket (especially for older children), if ordered.

6. Use icebags to promote comfort (but not for infants because this may cause chilling).

7. Observe the young child for seizures.

Cold water or alcohol baths are not used for the child. The cold water produces vasoconstriction and shivering, which raises the central body temperature. Alcohol reduces the temperature too quickly and may lead to convulsions in the small child, and the fumes are toxic. If the child can have a tub bath, sit him in tepid water up to midthigh. Provide suitable toys for play and plan to bathe the child for 20 to 30 minutes. Sponging and splashing during play will keep enough water on the child's skin for cooling. A tub bath is less frightening than a sponge bath, for which the child is covered with wet towels. If the child cannot be placed in the tub, a sponge bath may be given. Again, use tepid water.

Equipment

Plastic sheet
Two bath blankets
Hot water bottle with cover

Towels
Six washcloths or four-inch gauze squares
Tepid water

Procedure A

1. Give antipyretic drug (as ordered) 20 minutes before starting sponge bath to enhance effects of the bath.
2. Take temperature, pulse, and respirations before proceeding to provide a baseline for comparison to determine effectiveness of treatment.
3. Place plastic sheet, then bath blanket, under the child.
4. Undress the child and cover with second bath blanket.
5. Place hot water bottle at child's feet to help prevent chills and shivering.
6. Remove padding from inside gauze squares.
7. Open squares and soak in tepid water.
8. Place opened squares on abdomen, wrists, and ankles.
9. Rewet gauze every few minutes. Continue for 15 to 20 minutes.
10. Pat child dry with towel and dress him in lightweight clothes.
11. Recheck temperature in 30 minutes.

This procedure brings a temperature down more quickly than conventional sponging (procedure B).

Procedure B

Follow steps 1 through 5 of procedure A, then proceed as follows:

6. Wet washcloths in tepid water, wring slightly, then place on groin and each axilla.
7. Expose body part to be sponged; place a towel under the body part.
8. Using gentle friction to bring the blood to the surface, slowly stroke with wet washcloth. Stroke arm from neck to palm; stroke leg from groin to foot. Bathe back and buttocks.
9. Continue to sponge for 20 to 30 minutes unless the child becomes chilled or if cyanosis or mottling of the skin does not cease with gentle friction. If child begins to shiver, cover him and wait a few minutes.
10. Pat child dry with towel and dress him in lightweight clothes.
11. Recheck temperature in 30 minutes.

NEUROLOGIC STATUS ASSESSMENT

A neurologic status check, referred to as neurological danger orders or neurosurgic danger orders in different institutions, is a set of criteria for assessing the patient's neurologic condition. The criteria should be clearly stated so that each person using them knows exactly what they mean; otherwise, assessing and recording will be inconsistent. An example of a workable set of criteria is offered in Table 1-3.

Table 1-3 **Neurologic Check List**

Date	Time	B/P	T	P	R	Patent Airway	Level of Consciousness	Pupil Reaction and Eye Movement
	7							
	8							
	9							
	10							
	11							
	12							
	1							
	2							
	3							
	4							
	5							
	6							
	7							

NOTE: Patient NPO unless otherwise ordered. Check every hour unless otherwise ordered.

Notify MD of:

Pulse changes:	Full-term newborn	↓ 90 or ↑ 190
	Infant	↓ 75 or ↑ 175
	1–6 years	↓ 70 or ↑ 140
	6–12 years	↓ 65 or ↑ 125
	12–18 years	↓ 60 or ↑ 110

Respirations: any irregular pattern.
Blood pressure: any rise over child's baseline.
Temperature: ↑ 38.8°C (102°F)

Reaction to Verbal Stimuli	Reaction to Painful Stimuli	Muscular Response Strength	Reflexes	Signature

*Turn page for checklist code

Figure 1-24.

Neurologic Check List Code

Level of Consciousness

1. **Alert.** Fully aware of surroundings; oriented to time, place, person. Appropriate response to auditory, visual, motor, and sensory stimuli. (For a child, you must know his normal responses; play "peek-a-boo" or "patty cake" with him. If he is afraid, let his mother interact with him.)

2. **Obtunded.** Responds slowly or incompletely when stimulated, otherwise appears drowsy and indifferent, confused (dazed and disoriented), and delirious (uncooperative, easily agitated).

3. **Stuporous.** Responds after repeated vigorous stimuli. When aroused, is not oriented to time, place, and person.

4. **Coma.** Responds to painful stimuli with decorticate posturing (arms, wrists, and fingers flexed and clutched to body; legs extended, plantor flexed and internally rotated) or decerebrate posturing (opisthotonoid, clenched teeth; arms adducted and hyperpronated; legs stiffly extended).

5. **Deep coma.** No response to painful stimuli. No deep tendon, corneal, cough, or gag reflexes.

Pupillary Response

E/R Equal and react to light; otherwise measure reaction using descriptive terms such as sluggish, brisk, and so on.

L Left

R Right

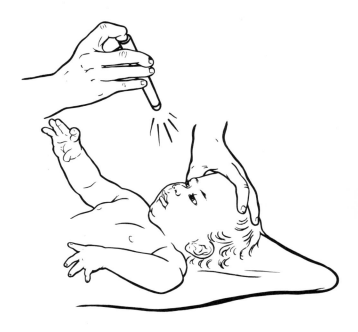

Check pupillary reaction to light by shining a penlight into pupil at a slight angle (Figure 1-24). Check both eyes.

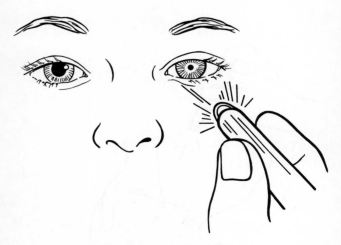

Figure 1-25.

Note response, whether equal and reactive (both eyes react to light equally) or sluggish, brisk, and so on (Figure 1-25). Terms such as *pinpoint*, *moderate*, and *dilated* cannot be interpreted consistently and should be avoided. A more accurate means of assessment is to measure the size of the pupil, using a chart of pupil sizes for reference. ECG paper can be used to make such a chart; the small squares are 1 millimeter and the large squares are 5 millimeters.

Eye Movement

Light coma. Doll's eye sign—when head is turned briskly, eyes roll in opposite direction.
Deep coma. Motionless, slightly divergent (in position of rest)

Muscular Strength
Test each extremity for paralysis, strength, and equal movement.

LA   Left arm
RA   Right arm
LL   Left leg
RL   Right leg

Reflexes
Test cough, swallow, and gag reflexes.

Babinski response.   Stroke sole of foot with pointed object from heel to ball, then across foot medially. Babinski response consists of fanning and dorsiflexion of toes in patients over 12 to 18 months of age and indicates neurologic dysfunction.

The following are signs of meningeal irritation:

Brudzinski's sign.   With child supine, passively flex his neck; if Brudzinski's sign is present, he will involuntarily flex his knees.
Kernig's sign.   Flex child's hip by raising his leg, then attempt to straighten the knee. If Kernig's sign is present, knee will not straighten and child will experience pain and muscle spasm.
Nuchal rigidity.   Stiff neck.

BIBLIOGRAPHY

Brunner, L.S. and Suddarth, D.S. *The Lippincott Manual of Nursing Practice*, ed 2. New York, JB Lippincott Co., 1978, pp. 1373–1379.

Chow, M.P.S., Durand, B.A., Feldman, M.N., et al. *Handbook of Pediatric Primary Care*. New York, John Wiley & Sons, 1979, p. 552.

Dower, J.C. Assessment and Care of the Child, in Rudolph, A.M. (ed). *Pediatrics*, ed 16. New York, Appleton-Century-Crofts, 1977, p. 52.

Fochtman, D. and Raffensperger, J.G. *Principles of Nursing Care For the Pediatric Surgery Patient*, ed 2. Boston, Little, Brown & Co., 1976, p. 3.

Johnson, T.R., Moore, W.M., Jeffries, J.E. *Children Are Different: Developmental Physiology*, ed. 2, Columbus, Ohio, Ross Laboratories, 1978, p 136.

Lieberman, E. Hypertension in Childhood and Adolescence, in *Clinical Symposia*, vol. 30. Summit, N.J., CIBA Pharmaceutical Company, 1978, pp. 3–9.

Marshall, F. Tips and Timesavers: Pupil Paper. *Nursing '78* 8:104, 1978.

McFarlane, J., Whitson, B.J., and Hartley, L.M. *Contemporary Pediatric Nursing: A Conceptual Approach*. New York, John Wiley & Sons, 1980.

Sundman, C. Quick-Cooling Gauze: Tips and Timesavers. *Nursing '79* 9:86, 1979.

The National Heart, Lung, and Blood Pressure Institute's Task Force on Blood Pressure Control in Children: Report of the Task Force on Blood Pressure Control in Children. *Pediatrics* 59 (suppl.):797–820, 1977.

CHAPTER **2**

Hygienic Needs of the Child

BATHING

Bathing is an important part of the child's daily routine. Avoid drafts and chilling. A comfortable room temperature is 23.9° to 26.7°C (75° to 80° F). Bath water should be 36.7° to 40.5° C (98° to 105° F) or warm to the antecubital fossa.

Bathing is done before, not after, a feeding to prevent vomiting or spitting up. Bathing begins at the cleanest part of the child's body and proceeds to the dirtiest; that is, from eyes and face to trunk, extremities, and genitals. If the newborn's cord has not fallen off (usually by 7 to 10 days), he should be given a sponge bath and not immersed in water. A wet cord remains in place longer and may become infected. Fingernails are cleaned and cut, if necessary, before the bath.

For a sponge bath, uncover only the area to be bathed. Wash, rinse, and dry the area before proceeding to the next body part. The genitals are washed in the same way whether the child is immersed or sponged. Even for a tub or basin bath, it is not necessary to undress the child until after the hair and face have been washed and dried. Although the illustrations in this chapter show an infant being bathed, the procedures are the same for an older child.

Equipment

To avoid undue exposure, assemble the following equipment before undressing the child:

Basin (for sponge or bed bath) or sink or tub (for immersion bath)
Soft washcloth
Three towels
Mild soap
Clean diaper and shirt (or underpants and pajamas for the older child)
Hairbrush

Ointments and powders are normally not used; however, the physician may prescribe a soothing lotion for dry skin.

Procedure for Bathing

Hold the child's head securely with one hand; with the other hand, wipe gently from the inner canthus outward (Figure 2-1). Use only clear water, no soap. Wipe the other eye with a clean portion of the washcloth to prevent the possible spread of any infection.

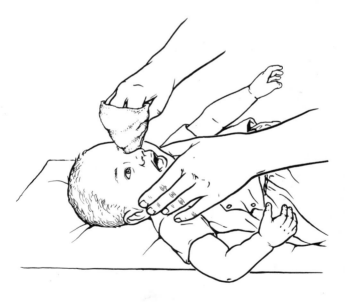

Figure 2-1.

Gently wash the outer ear and external canal with one finger inside the washcloth (Figure 2-2). Do not use cotton-tipped applicators because they may injure the ear.

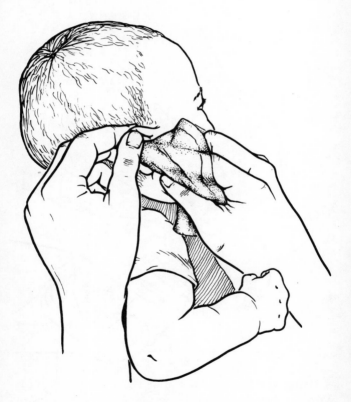

Figure 2-2.

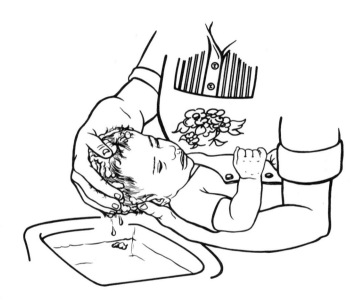

Figure 2-3.

Using the football hold (p. 181), lather the hair
with one hand and gently massage the head (Figure
2-3). Avoid getting soap in the eyes. If the child is

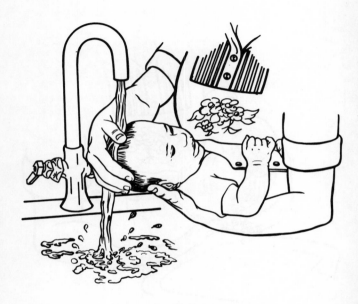

Figure 2-4A

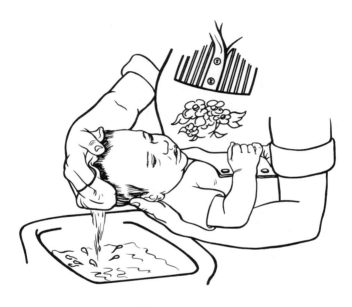

Figure 2-4B

bathed at the sink, rinse his hair under slow-running water (Figure 2-4A). If the child is bathed at the beside, rinse his hair over the basin, using a washcloth (Figure 2-4B). Dry hair thoroughly.

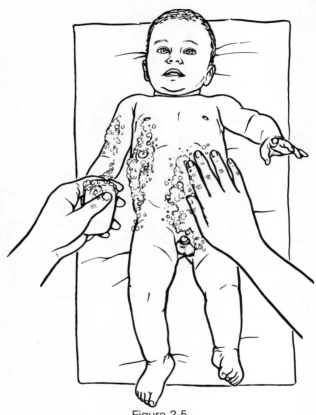

Figure 2-5.

The following procedures are for the infant or child who can be immersed in a sink or basin: Undress the infant and place him on a towel. Lather the trunk and extremities with your hands, making sure to wash all skin creases (Figure 2-5).

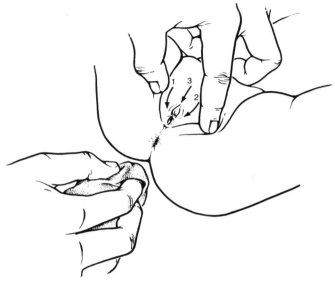

Figure 2-6.

For girls, separate the labia with one hand and wash from front to back (in the order indicated by arrows in Figure 2-6) to prevent infection of vagina and/or urethra with fecal material.

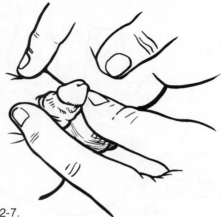

Figure 2-7.

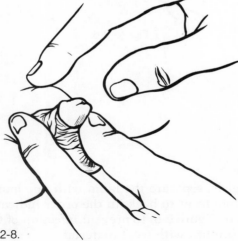

Figure 2-8.

For the circumcised boy, gently wash the penis and scrotum (Figure 2-7).

For the uncircumcised boy, retract the foreskin of the penis and cleanse (Figure 2-8). Daily retraction and cleansing prevents penile adhesions.

Remember that the soapy child is slippery; use the utmost care when picking him up (Figure 2-9). Dry your hands; then firmly pick him up and place him in basin or sink.

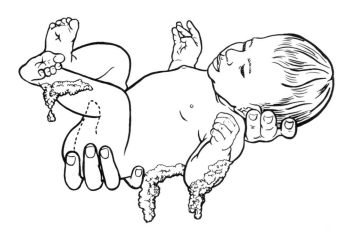

Figure 2-9.

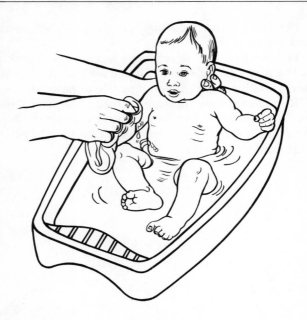

Figure 2-10.

Support the child's head with one hand, and use a washcloth in your other hand to rinse him (Figure 2-10). If a sink is used, place a towel in the bottom to stabilize the child and avoid slipping. Because exercise and water play are important and stimulating to the child's development, allow him to play and splash in the water if his condition permits.

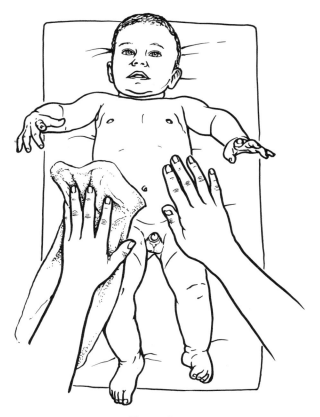

Figure 2-11.

Remove the child from the basin or sink and place him on a clean towel for drying (Figure 2-11).

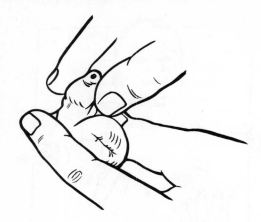

Figure 2-12.

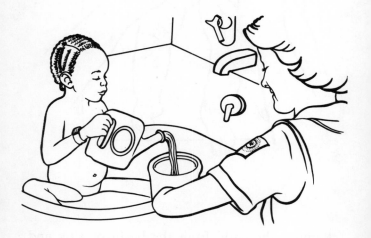

Figure 2-13.

Replace the retracted foreskin on the uncircumcised boy to prevent paraphimosis (Figure 2-12). Dress the child appropriately.

When bathing the older child in a tub, stay with him to assure his safety (Figure 2-13). Provide plastic or sponge toys and permit water play if his condition allows. Fifteen to 30 minutes is usually sufficient for a bath and water play and will not cause chilling.

DIAPERING

Procedure

Cloth diapers may be folded in a triangle (Figure 2-14A) or a rectangle (Figure 2-14B). When using the rectangular fold, place the extra thickness at the back for girls and in the front for boys.

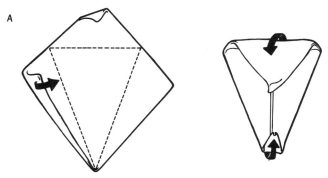

Figure 2-14 A

B

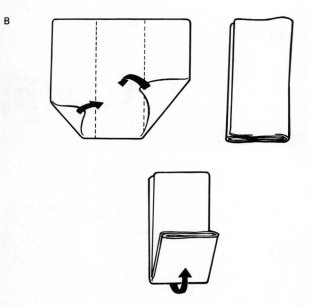

Figure 2-14B

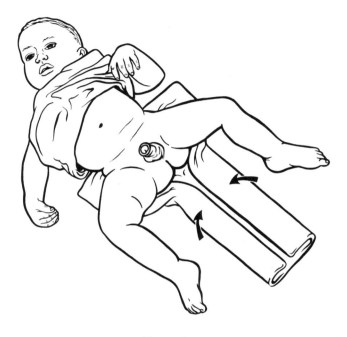

Figure 2-15.

Place the diaper under the infant's buttocks and fold sides in, between his legs (Figure 2-15). This keeps bulk of diaper in perineal area to contain the urine and feces and does not restrict leg movement.

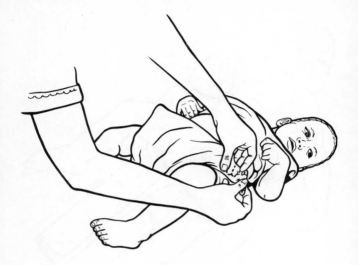

Figure 2-16.

Bring diaper up over abdomen; place front part of diaper next to baby's skin; bring back of diaper over front and pin, being careful to place your finger between the baby and the diaper to avoid sticking him (Figure 2-16). (During the diaper change, close the pins and place them out of the infant's reach.)

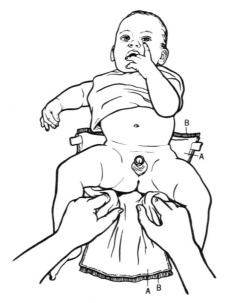

Figure 2-17.

A disposable diaper (Figure 2-17) consists of an inner layer of absorbent material (A) and an outer layer of plastic (B). The plastic overlaps the absorbent material by about an inch at the front and back of the diaper. Fold this excess in before securing the diaper; otherwise, the absorbent material (which acts like a wick) will come in contact with the infant's clothing or linen and wet it. If the infant is allergic to the plastic, fold the absorbent material out over the plastic. (Cloth diapers may be preferable to disposable for the allergic child.)

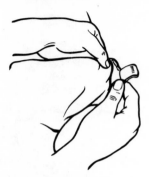

Figure 2-18.

Place the front of the diaper next to the infant's skin and bring the back portion (with the adhesive tab attached) over the front and secure (Figure 2-18).

CHAPTER 3

The Child's Growth Needs

MEASUREMENTS

Measurable growth, evidenced by height (or length), weight, and head and chest circumference, is one of the chief characteristics that distinguishes children from adults. These routine measurements, particularly height and weight, provide an overall measure of the child's growth as well as a record for comparison with the norm on standard growth charts.

Height

Equipment

Yardstick (or measuring board for infants).
Paper tape measure (cloth or plastic stretch with use and may not be accurate)
Wall measuring board (or standard scales with height measure for older child)

Procedure for Measuring Height

Place the infant on flat surface with heel of foot

perpendicular to and even with edge of yardstick or measuring board (Figure 3-1). With one hand, hold the infant's leg straight; with the other hand, mark crown of head against measure. If no measuring board or yardstick is available, mark the exact spot on the paper or sheet where the infant's heel and crown rest with a pencil; then measure this length and record.

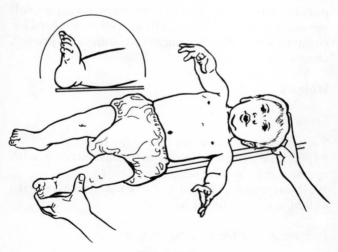

Figure 3-1.

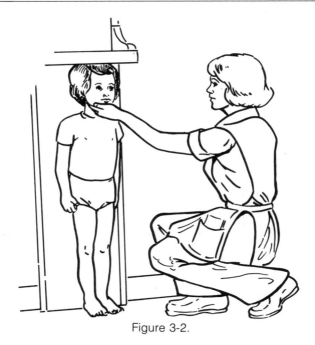

Figure 3-2.

When the child can stand erect, measure him on a wall measuring board, if one is available (Figure 3-2). Have him stand erect, with back, head, and heels touching the wall. Hold his head steady and lower horizontal bar to level of head. Record measurement.

To measure a child on an adult scale (Figure 3-3), have the child stand erect with heels, back, and head touching the vertical portion of scale. The horizontal bar is lowered to meet head. Record height.

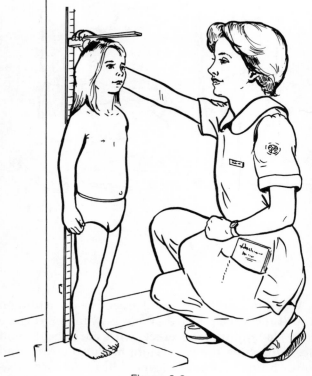

Figure 3-3.

Weight

Equipment

Infant scales for child under one year of age; paper liners
Adult scales for the older child

Procedure for Measuring Weight

Place a paper liner on infant scale (Figure 3-4). Adjust scale if necessary so it is balanced. Put the naked infant on scale, keeping one hand close to but not touching the baby to prevent his falling. Apply

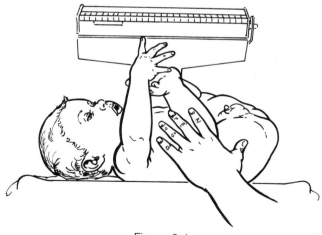

Figure 3-4.

weights or move weight bar until scale balances. After weighing, discard the paper liner and return weights to zero position. Record weight.

Place a paper liner on scale and adjust if necessary so scale is balanced (Figure 3-5). Have the child stand still while you adjust weights. The child

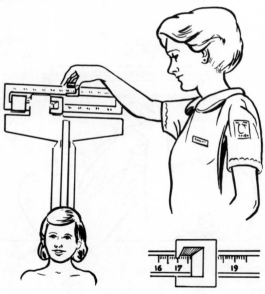

Figure 3-5.

may wear street clothes or pajamas but no shoes, heavy sweaters, or coats. If the child cannot or will not stand still to be weighed, let another adult hold him while you weigh them both. Weigh the adult separately, then subtract this weight from the combined weight; this gives you the child's weight, although it is not as accurate as weighing the child alone. The child shown in Figure 3-5 weighs 17 kilograms.

Head and Chest Circumference

Head and chest circumferences are checked on all children under two years of age. They are not routinely checked on the child over that age. At birth, the average head circumference will measure 34 to 37 centimeters (13 to 14½ inches). The chest measures about 2 centimeters less. Disproportionate head measurements may indicate hydrocephaly or microcephaly; the chest may be large or small. Until two years of age, these two measures are approximately the same, with the head being slightly larger. After age two, the chest size increases more rapidly than does the head.

Equipment

Paper tape measure

Procedure for Measuring Head and Chest

Measure head at greatest circumference with a paper tape (Figure 3-6). Measure chest at nipple line and record both measurements.

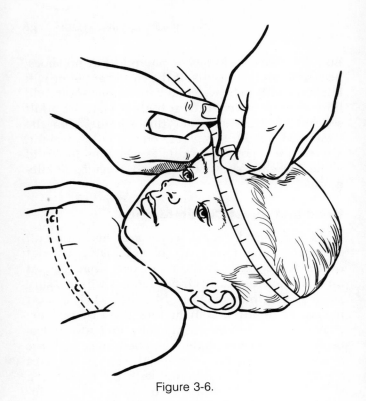

Figure 3-6.

Growth Grids

Length, weight, and, sometimes, head circumference are plotted against the child's chronologic age on standardized growth grids. Measurements between the 25th and 75th percentiles usually indicate normal growth. Measurements between the 10th and 25th or 75th and 90th percentiles may indicate either normal growth or a deviation. Factors such as the child's past and future measurements, general health, family stature, dietary patterns, and developmental milestones must be considered when evaluating the child's standing in relation to growth percentiles. Measurements below the 10th and above the 90th percentiles are considered suspicious; those under the 5th and over the 95th percentiles are a cause for concern and are further evaluated. Children under the 10th percentile may be suffering from failure-to-thrive; those over the 95th are usually obese. Any child whose measurements change by more than 20 percentiles is carefully assessed for possible problems.

Although growth grids are available for boys and girls of various ages, only one grid is presented here with instructions for plotting the length and weight.

Procedure for Plotting Growth Grids

Growth grid—Girls: Birth to 36 months (Figure 3-7). (Adapted from the National Center for Health Statistics: NCHS Growth Charts, 1976. *Monthly Vital Statistics Report* 25;3 (Supp) [HRA] 76–1120. Data from The Fels Research Institute, Yellow Springs, Ohio. Charts prepared by Ross Laboratories, Columbus, Ohio, 1976.)

Kelly, twenty-one months old, weighs 11.6 kilograms (25½ pounds) and is 84 centimeters (33¼ inches) long. Plotted on the growth grid, her weight is in the 55th percentile (A) and her length is in the 50th percentile (B). Both are within normal limits.

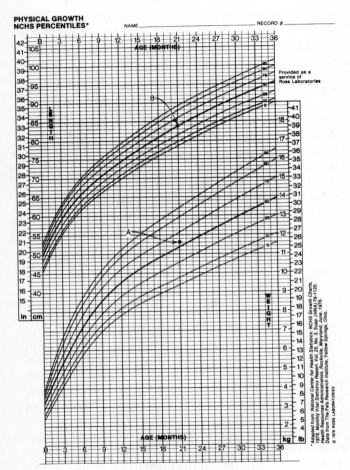

Figure 3-7.

DEVELOPMENTAL ASSESSMENT

Developmental screening tests are useful as simple tools to determine if the child should be referred for more extensive examination for developmental delay. However, brief screening tests bring with them a certain amount of error. A normal child, for instance, may be falsely identified as retarded if the test includes evaluation of a skill in which he is not particularly strong. Another child may draw a human figure with ease but may suffer from a serious language handicap that produces a specific learning disability. For these reasons, screening tools are *not* considered diagnostic; rather, they are used to *screen* children who may need further evaluation.

The tests included in this book are easily administered and have demonstrated reliability.

Goodenough-Harris Draw-a-Person Test

Used for children between three and thirteen years of age. It measures IQ and offers insight into child's self-concept and emotions.

Procedure for Administering

Give child a No. 2 pencil with eraser and a blank sheet of paper. Ask him to "draw a person; draw the best person you can." No additional instructions are needed; however, encouragement may be given if necessary. Do not suggest that the child's drawing be changed or supplemented in any way, unless he has drawn a stick figure. In this case, ask him to "draw a whole person."

Scoring: Using the scoring guides in Tables 3-1 and 3-2. Give one point for each detail present. Minimum score for the child should be within one standard deviation of mean for age.

Table 3-1. **Details Present**

Drawing of a Man

1. Head present
2. Neck present
3. Neck, two dimensions
4. Eyes present
5. Eye detail: brow or lashes
6. Eye detail: pupil
7. Nose present
8. Nose, two dimensions (not round ball)
9. Mouth present
10. Lips, two dimensions
11. Both nose and lips in two dimensions
12. Both chin and forehead shown
13. Bridge of nose (straight to eyes; narrower than base)
14. Hair I (any scribble)
15. Hair II (more detail)
16. Ears present
17. Fingers present
18. Correct number of fingers shown
19. Opposition of thumb shown (must include fingers)
20. Hands present
21. Arms present
22. Arms at side or engaged in activity
23. Feet: any indication
24. Attachment of arms and legs I (to trunk anywhere)
25. Attachment of arms and legs II (at correct point of trunk)
26. Trunk present
27. Trunk in proportion, two dimensions (length greater than breadth)
28. Clothing I (anything)
29. Clothing II (2 articles of clothing)

Table 3-1.   (continued)

Drawing of a Woman

1. Head present
2. Neck present
3. Neck, two dimensions
4. Eyes present
5. Eye detail: brow or lashes
6. Eye detail: pupil
7. Nose present (not round ball)
8. Nose, two dimensions
9. Bridge of nose (straight to eyes, narrower than base)
10. Nostrils shown
11. Mouth present
12. Lips, two dimensions
13. Both nose and lips in two dimensions
14. Both chin and forehead shown
15. Hair I (any scribble)
16. Hair II (more detail)
17. Necklace or earrings
18. Arms present
19. Fingers present
20. Correct number of fingers shown
21. Opposition of thumb shown (must include fingers)
22. Hands present
23. Legs present
24. Feet (any indication)
25. Shoe "feminine" (any attempt such as high heels, open toe, strap)
26. Attachment of arms and legs I (to trunk anywhere)
27. Attachment of arms and legs II (to trunk at correct point)
28. Clothing indicated (any)
29. Sleeve
30. Neckline (any indication)
31. Trunk present
32. Trunk in proportion, two dimensions (length greater than breadth)

Table 3-2. Scoring

| | Drawing of Man | | Drawing of Woman | |
Age	By Boys	By Girls	By Boys	By Girls
3	4	5	4	6
4	7	7	7	8
5	11	12	11	14
6	13	14	13	16
7	16	17	16	19
8	18	20	20	23

Reproduced with permission from Johns Hopkins Hospital: *The Harriet Lane Handbook*, Ed. 8.   Kenneth C. Schuberth and Basil J. Zitelli (Eds). Copyright © 1978 by Year Book Medical Publishers, Inc., Chicago.

Developmental Milestones

Table 3-3 presents a list of achievements and milestones that most parents will remember and that emphasize language skills.

Table 3-3. Developmental Assessment

Age	Gross Motor	Visual Motor	Language	Social
1 month	Raises head slightly from prone, makes crawling movements	Has tight grasp, follows to midline	Alerts to sound (e.g. by blinking, moving, startling)	Regards face
2 months	Holds head in midline	No longer clenches fist tightly, follows object past midline	Smiles after being stroked or talked to	Acts increasingly alert
3 months	Supports on forearms in prone, holds head up steadily	Holds hands open at rest, pulls at clothing	Coos (produces long vowel sounds in musical fashion)	Reaches for familiar people or objects, anticipates feeding
4 months	Sits well when propped	Moves arms in unison to graps. touches cube placed on table	Orients to voice 5 mos – turns head toward bell, says "ah-goo"	Enjoys looking around environment

Table 3-3. Developmental Assessment (continued)

Age	Gross Motor	Visual Motor	Language	Social
6 months	Rolls from back to front, sits well, puts feet in mouth in supine position	Reaches with either hand, transfers, uses raking grasp	Babbles *7 mos*—waves bye-bye *8 mos*—"dada/mama" inappropriately	Recognizes strangers, plays pat-a-cake
9 months	Creeps, pulls to feet, likes to stand	Uses overhand pincer grasp, probes with forefinger, holds bottle, finger-feeds	Imitates sounds *10 mos*—"dada/mama" appropriately *11 mos*—one word	Starts to explore environment
12 months	Walks alone or with hand held, pivots when sitting, cooperates with dressing	Uses pincer grasp, throws objects, lets go of toys	Follows one-step command with gesture, uses two words *14 mos*—uses three words	Imitates actions, comes when called, cooperates with dressing
15 months	Walks well, creeps	Builds tower of 2	Follows one-step	

Age	Gross motor	Fine motor	Language	Social
		of examiner, scribbles in imitation	gesture, uses 4-6 words and immature jargoning (runs several unintelligible words together)	Copies parent in tasks (e.g. sweeping, dusting), plays in company of other children
18 months	Runs, throws toy from standing without falling	Turns 2 to 3 pages at a time, fills spoon and feeds himself	Knows 7 to 20 words, points to one body part when named, uses mature jargoning (includes intelligible words in jargoning)	Asks to have food and to go to toilet
21 months	Squats in play, goes up steps	Builds tower of 5 blocks, drinks well from cup	Points to 3 body parts, uses two-word combinations, points to 5 body parts	
24 months	Walks up and down steps without help	Turns pages one at a time, removes shoes, pants, etc.	Uses 50 words, two-word sentences, and three pronouns, names objects in pictures	

Table 3-3. Developmental Assessment (continued)

Age	Gross Motor	Visual Motor	Language	Social
2 years	Jumps, with both feet off floor, throws ball overhand	Unbuttons, holds pencil in adult fashion	Uses plurals, past tense and pronoun "I" correctly most of the time	Tells first and last name when asked, gets himself drink without help
3 years	Pedals tricycle, can alternate feet when going up steps	Dresses and undresses partially, dries hands if reminded	Tells story about experiences, knows his/her sex	Shares toys, takes turns, plays well with others
4 years	Hops, skips, alternates feet going downstairs	Buttons clothing fully, catches ball	Knows all colors, says song or poem from memory	Tells "tall tales," plays cooperatively with a group of children
5 years	Skips, alternating feet, jumps over low obstacles	Ties shoes, spreads with knife	Prints first name, asks what a word means	Plays competitive games, abides by rules, likes to help in household tasks

Reproduced with permission from Johns Hopkins Hospital: *The Harriet Lane Handbook*, Ed. 8. Kenneth C. Schuberth and Basil J. Zitelli (Eds). Copyright © 1978 by Year Book Medical Publishers, Inc., Chicago.

Denver Developmental Screening Test

The Denver Developmental Screening Test (DDST) is used for screening children from birth to six years of age. It encompasses four categories of development: personal-social, fine motor-adaptive, language, and gross motor. Specific instructions are included in the test manual, and the examiner must be trained in the use of the test. The test sheet itself is shown on the following pages for quick reference (Figure 3-8).

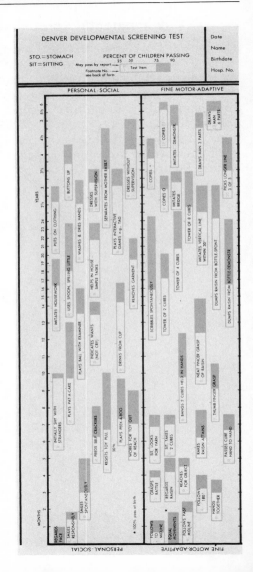

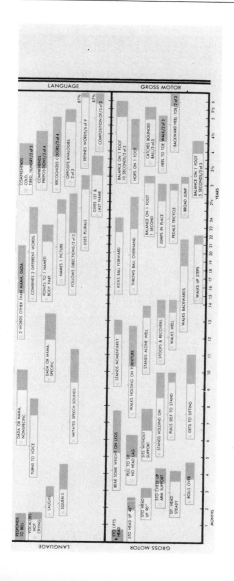

Figure 3-8A

| DIRECTIONS | DATE | BIRTHDATE |
| | NAME | HOSP. NO. |

1. Try to get child to smile by smiling, talking or waving to him. Do not touch him.
2. When child is playing with toy, pull it away from him. Pass if he resists.
3. Child does not have to be able to tie shoes or button in the back.
4. Move yarn slowly in an arc from one side to the other, about 6" above child's face.
   Pass if eyes follow 90° to midline. (Past midline; 180°)
5. Pass if child grasps rattle when it is touched to the backs or tips of fingers.
6. Pass if child continues to look where yarn disappeared or tries to see where it went. Yarn should be dropped quickly from sight from tester's hand without arm movement.
7. Pass if child picks up raisin with any part of thumb and a finger.
8. Pass if child picks up raisin with the ends of thumb and index finger using an over hand approach.

9. Pass any enclosed form. Fail continuous round motions.
10. Which line is longer? (Not bigger.) Turn paper upside down and repeat. (3/3 or 5/6)
11. Pass any crossing lines.
12. Have child copy first. If failed, demonstrate

When giving items 9, 11 and 12, do not name the forms. Do not demonstrate 9 and 11.

13. When scoring, each pair (2 arms, 2 legs, etc.) counts as one part.
14. Point to picture and have child name it. (No credit is given for sounds only.)

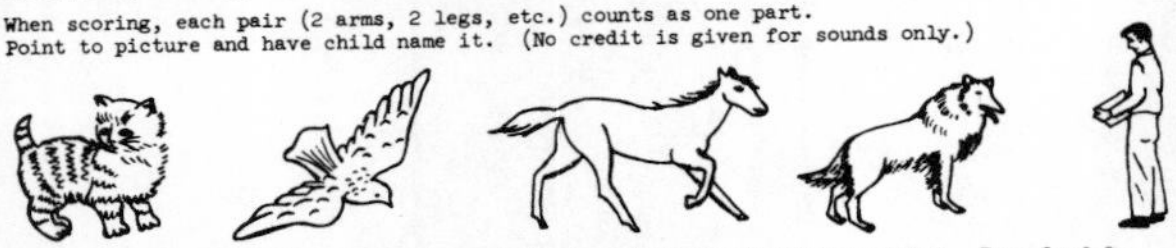

15. Tell child to: Give block to Mommie; put block on table; put block on floor. Pass 2 of 3. (Do not help child by pointing, moving head or eyes.)
16. Ask child: What do you do when you are cold? ..hungry? ..tired? Pass 2 of 3.
17. Tell child to: Put block on table; under table; in front of chair, behind chair. Pass 3 of 4. (Do not help child by pointing, moving head or eyes.)
18. Ask child: If fire is hot, ice is ?; Mother is a woman, Dad is a ?; a horse is big, a mouse is ?. Pass 2 of 3.
19. Ask child: What is a ball? ..lake? ..desk? ..house? ..banana? ..curtain? ..ceiling? ..hedge? ..pavement? Pass if defined in terms of use, shape, what it is made of or general category (such as banana is fruit, not just yellow). Pass 6 of 9.
20. Ask child: What is a spoon made of? ..a shoe made of? ..a door made of? (No other objects may be substituted.) Pass 3 of 3.
21. When placed on stomach, child lifts chest off table with support of forearms and/or hands.
22. When child is on back, grasp his hands and pull him to sitting. Pass if head does not hang back.
23. Child may use wall or rail only, not person. May not crawl.
24. Child must throw ball overhand 3 feet to within arm's reach of tester.
25. Child must perform standing broad jump over width of test sheet. (8-1/2 inches)
26. Tell child to walk forward, ⊂⊃⊂⊃⊂⊃⊂⊃► heel within 1 inch of toe. Tester may demonstrate. Child must walk 4 consecutive steps, 2 out of 3 trials.
27. Bounce ball to child who should stand 3 feet away from tester. Child must catch ball with hands, 2 out of 3 trials.
28. Tell child to walk backward, ◄⊂⊃⊂⊃⊂⊃⊂⊃ toe within 1 inch of heel. Tester may demonstrate. Child must walk 4 consecutive steps, 2 out of 3 trials.

DATE AND BEHAVIORAL OBSERVATIONS (how child feels at time of test, relation to tester, attention span, verbal behavior, self-confidence, etc,):

Figure 3-8 B

FEEDING TECHNIQUES

After feedings, chart the type and amount of nourishment taken and how the child tolerated the feeding.

Infant

Bottle Feeding
Get comfortable, have the bottle within easy reach; hold the infant securely in your arms and be sure

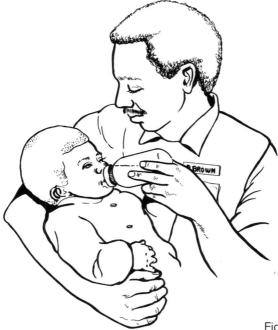

Figure 3-9.

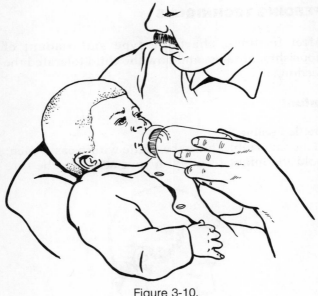

Figure 3-10.

that liquid covers hole in nipple to prevent the infant from swallowing air (Figure 3-9).

In Figure 3-10, the bottle is held incorrectly; the infant is swallowing air as well as formula. (The infant also may be fed solids while being held in the arms.)

Solids

The infant may be fed solids while seated in an infant seat (Figure 3-11). Note that he is strapped in for safety. He also has a spoon to hold during feedings; this is a developmental aid, intended to encourage the association of the spoon, which the child will eventually use himself, with feedings.

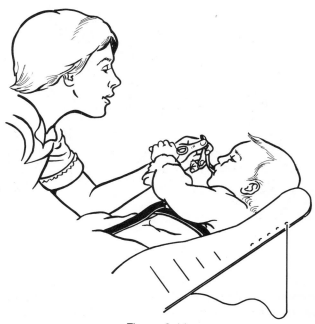

Figure 3-11.

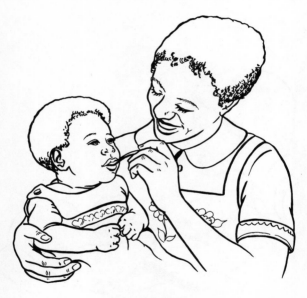

Figure 3-12.

When the infant is old enough to sit alone, he may be fed sitting on the adult's lap rather than in an infant seat (Figure 3-12). Note that the nurse's arm is around his back for support.

Child

The young child may sit in a high chair to eat (Figure 3-13). A safety strap is used to prevent falling.

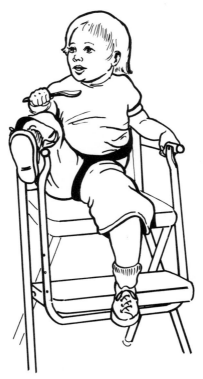

Figure 3-13.

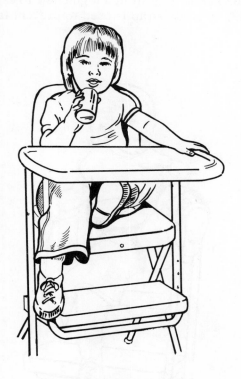

Figure 3-14.

With the tray attached to the high chair, the child
has his own "table" (Figure 3-14).

Burping

The bottle-fed newborn may need to be burped after every ½ to 1 ounce of formula (the breast-fed baby does not swallow as much air and does not need to be burped as frequently).

Procedure for Burping

Seat the infant on your lap, supporting his head by placing your hand on his chin, *not* on his neck, as he leans forward slightly (Figure 3-15). Gently pat his back or rub it from waist to shoulders until he burps. Continue feeding.

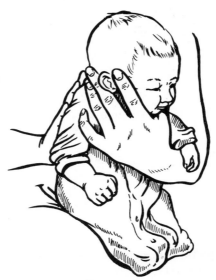

Figure 3-15.

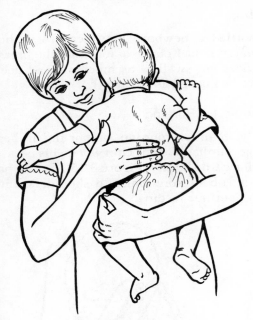

Figure 3-16.

Place the infant upright so that he is looking over your shoulder (Figure 3-16). Gently pat his back until he burps.

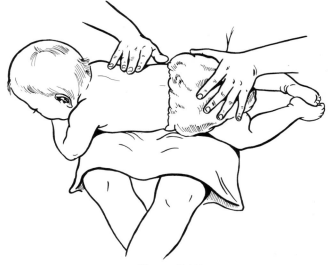

Figure 3-17.

An older infant may be placed across your lap (Figure 3-17). Prevent his falling with one hand and pat his back with the other until he burps.

See Table 3-4 for a list of common oral solutions and their nutritional values.

Table 3-4. Composition of Frequently Used Oral Solutions

Liquid	CHO gm/100ml	Prot.* gm/100ml	Cal/L	Na	K	Cl	HCO₃₃₁₁ mEq/L††	Ca	P†
Apple juice	14.3	—	522	1.9	26.6	—	—	—	—
Coca Cola	10.9	—	435	0.4	13	—	13.4	—	—
Gatorade	4.7	—	181	21	2.5	17	—	—	—
Ginger ale	9.0	—	360	3.5	0.1	—	3.6	2.7	—
Grape juice	18.0	—	670	0.4	31	—	32	—	—
Jell-O Water (1/2 strength)	8.0	0.8	338	5.5-16.5‡	0.1-0.2‡	—	—	—	—
Kool-aid (unsweetened)‡‡	—	6	—	0.2	0.1	—	—	—	—
Lytren	7.0	—	280	25	25	30	18	4	5
Milk (skim)	5.5	3.5	375	23	43	29	—	62	57
Milk (whole)	4.9	3.5	670	22	36	28	30	60	54

Orange juice (sweetened)	14.0	—	540	0.2	49	—	30	—	50	—	0
Pedialyte	5.0	—	200	30	20	—	—	14	4	0
Pepsi-Cola	12.0	—	480	6.5	0.8	—	—	7.3	—	8
R.C. Cola	10.5	—	421	0.07	0.04	—	—	—	—	
7-UP	10.15	—	411	7.0	0.5	—	—	—	5.0	—
Water (Baltimore City)	—	—	—	3	0.5	4	—	—	—	6.8

Reproduced with permission from Johns Hopkins Hospital: *The Harriet Lane Handbook*, ed. 8. Kenneth C. Schuberth and Basil J. Zitelli (eds). Copyright © 1978 by Year Book Medical Publishers, Inc., Chicago.

* Protein or amino acid equivalent

** Actual or potential bicarbonate, such as lactate, citrate or acetate

† Calculated according to valence of 1.8

†† Approximate values: actual values may vary somewhat in various localities depending on electrolyte composition of water supply used to reconstitute solution.

‡ Depends on flavor, (concord grape, black raspberry-lowest Na; wild cherry-highest Na)

‡‡ Does not include electrolyte contribution from local water

Special Feeding Techniques

Cleft Lip/Palate

The child with a cleft lip or palate may not be able to form a vacuum and therefore may be unable to suck. Several methods for feeding these children are offered below; others include the use of a *lamb's* nipple or "premie" nipple (both of these are soft and easier to suck), and a regular nipple with an enlarged hole. Be aware that the infant will cough, sputter, and choke during feedings and that the feeding will run back out of the cleft(s). Hold the infant upright to decrease risk of aspiration and to allow the cough reflex to clear his airway. Burp him often because he tends to swallow a lot of air.

A commercially available nurser with disposable bags to contain the formula may be used (Figure 3-18). Longitudinal slits are already cut into the hard plastic nurser to permit easy visualization of bag contents. Enlarge these slits with scissors or a knife so that your index finger will fit through the opening to compress the bag, or place index finger through open bottom of nurser and compress bag with finger. By compressing the bag as the infant sucks, you can ensure an adequate intake and at the same time control the amount of fluid to prevent choking and aspiration. In addition, the infant gains satisfaction from "sucking."

Feeding with a syringe and short length of tubing is less satisfactory than the above technique but may be necessary on occasion (Figure 3-19). This technique should be used before surgery for lip repair to accustom the infant to the way he will be fed

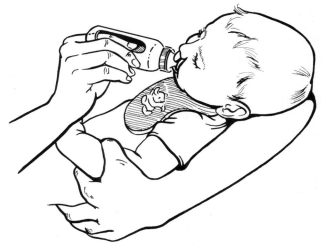

Figure 3-18.

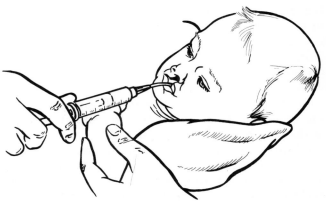

Figure 3-19.

postoperatively. Attach a short length of feeding tubing to a 10-cc syringe. Get comfortable, hold the infant "in arms," and keep his hands out of the way. Formula should be within easy reach. Fill a syringe to level that can be comfortably managed with one hand. Place the feeding tube to back and side of mouth and slowly squeeze formula into mouth, giving the infant time to swallow.

This technique is frustrating for the infant, especially if he is hungry because he cannot get enough fast enough. After he awakens from surgery, he is hungry and can usually be fed right away, provided no stress is placed on the suture line. (He is not permitted to suck and feeding with a medicine dropper is too slow for him). After feeding, always give clear water to wash formula from suture line.

Because the infant with a cleft palate cannot suck effectively, he is usually taught early to drink from a cup (Figure 3-20). After surgery for repair of the palate, nothing can be placed in the child's mouth (to prevent trauma to the suture line); therefore, if he has *not* been drinking from a cup at home, he is encouraged to do so before surgery to accustom him to the method of drinking that he will use postoperatively.

For feeding solids, use the *side* of a spoon so that the spoon itself does not enter the child's mouth; never use the end of the spoon. Rinse with clear water after feedings to clean the suture line.

To clean the suture line after a cleft-lip repair, use sterile cotton-tipped applicators and hydrogen peroxide (or sterile water) (Figure 3-21). Begin on one side of the suture line and gently roll the mois-

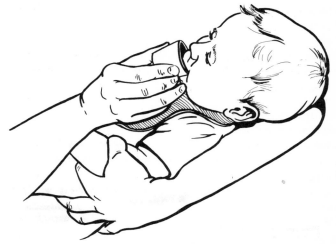

Figure 3-20.

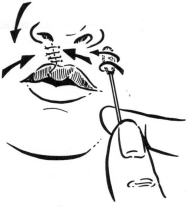

Figure 3-21.

tened applicator to the *middle* of the suture line. Discard applicator. Repeat for other side. Using a third moistened applicator, gently roll down from nares to lip and discard. Repeat these steps until the suture line is free of blood and crusts (which cause scarring). Gently clean the sutures inside the lip also.

Gavage Feedings
Nasogastric intubation may be necessary for gavage feedings or to decompress the stomach. A small-diameter, disposable, polyethylene catheter is preferred. The method of measurement is the same for oral or nasal insertion. Oral insertion causes less of a gag reflex, less chance of aspiration, and less irritation. Rolling the tubing into a circle before insertion will allow it to follow the contour of the nasopharynx into the stomach, thus making its passage easier.

During feedings, keep the child as quiet as possible to prevent regurgitation and aspiration. If he becomes active or restless during the feeding, stop the feeding until he quiets down; if he gags, coughs, or regurgitates, stop the feeding until the episode passes.

Equipment

Proper-size nasogastric tube:
   Premature infant—#3½ to 5 French
   Children—#8 to 10 French
   Adolescents—#12 to 14 French
Water-soluble lubricant

Towel
Cup of water
Stethoscope
20- to 50-cc syringe
Formula

Procedure for Gavage Feeding

For the infant and small child, measure from tip of nose to midpoint between xiphoid process and umbilicus. See Figure 3-22, A.

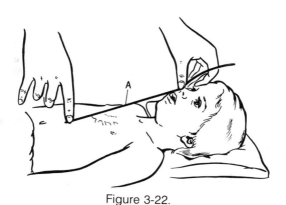

Figure 3-22.

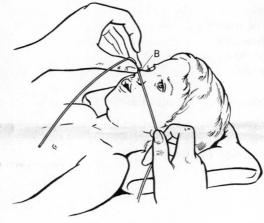

Figure 3-23.

Measure from tip of nose to lobe of ear (B, Figure 3-23). Add length of A and B, and mark total length on tubing with indelible pen or tape. (For the older child, measure from earlobe to bridge of nose to xiphoid.)

Wrap the infant snugly in a mummy restraint (see Chapter 5) and place him in a supine position. Give the older child a towel to cover his chest and a glass of water to drink with a straw (if permitted), or have him swallow during the insertion to facilitate passage. Hyperflex the neck and stabilize the head with one hand. With your other hand, quickly insert the catheter with a gentle twist. (Lubrication with water or water-soluble jelly is optional, since mucous secretions provide adequate lubrication.) If you meet with resistance, coughing, cyanosis, or choking, withdraw the catheter; let the child rest a few minutes, and reinsert.

After insertion, tape the catheter to the child's face where it leaves the nose. (see Figure 3-24). Do *not* tape it to his forehead because this places it against the tip of the nares and causes irritation and tissue breakdown.

Determine that tube has been correctly placed in the stomach, using at least two of the following three methods (see Figure 3-24). (*1*) Insert 0.5 to 1

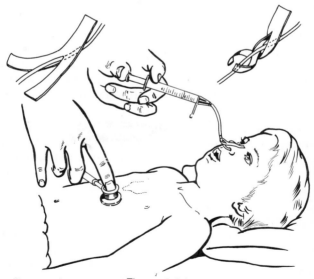

Figure 3-24.

milliliter air into the catheter and listen with a
stethoscope over the stomach for the rush of air (a
slight pop) into the stomach. (*2*) Withdraw a small
amount of stomach contents (then replace them).
(*3*) Put the open end of the catheter in a glass of
water while the child is exhaling (never while he is
inhaling)—bubbles will form continuously if the
catheter is misplaced in the trachea.

In order to avoid distention of the stomach in
premature infants, the amount of stomach aspirate
retained from the previous feeding is subtracted
from the amount to be given. Record amount aspirated.

Hold the child if possible; otherwise, place him
in supine position or turned slightly to the right
with a blanket roll behind his back (Figure 3-25).
Permit the infant to suck a pacifier during the feeding unless he is too weak or too sick to suck. Elevate
reservoir (usually a 20- to 50-cc syringe without the
plunger) about 15 to 20 centimeters (6 to 8 inches)
above child's head and allow feeding to flow in
slowly by gravity. Feeding too rapidly will cause
abdominal distension and regurgitation. Feeding
time should last as long as if the same amount was
fed by nipple. If the small lumen of the catheter
prolongs feeding time, gentle pressure may be
exerted at the rate of 3 cc/min, depending on the
size of the infant.

After feedings, clear the tubing with clear water,
using 5 cubic centimeters for premature infants, 10
cubic centimeters for infants, or an adequate
amount to flush the tubing. Pinch the tubing before

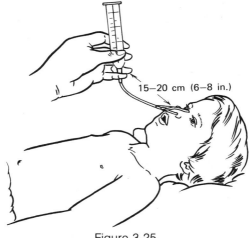

15—20 cm (6—8 in.)

Figure 3-25.

all the water reaches the end of the catheter and withdraw quickly. Clamping the end prevents air from entering the stomach and causing abdominal distention and also prevents formula from dripping into the pharynx, causing gagging and aspiration. If the tubing is to remain in place (never longer than 72 hours), the end is clamped. Burp the infant and leave him on his abdomen or right side. Accurately chart the procedure, type, and amount of feeding, amount of residual aspirate, amount of water used to clear tubing, how child tolerated the feeding, any vomiting, and child's activity after the feeding.

Gastrostomy Feeding

Gastrostomy tubes are used to decompress the stomach or to offer feedings if the child is unable to take nourishment orally. The tube is inserted surgically into the stomach through the abdominal wall and is held in place by sutures or tape.

Equipment

20- to 50-cc syringe
Sterile water
Warmed feeding or formula

Procedure for Gastrostomy Feeding

Tubing is attached to a 20- to 50-cc syringe for feedings. Hold the child if possible; otherwise, elevate his head and chest slightly (Figure 3-26). Elevate the syringe 10 to 12 centimeters (4 to 4¾ inches) and allow feeding to flow in by gravity. Never force the feeding. His condition permitting, the infant may be given a pacifier to suck during the feeding to help fulfill his sucking need, to relax him, and to help him equate the sucking reflex with the satisfaction of hunger.

After feedings, do *not* clamp tubing unless physician has so ordered. Tubing may be elevated after the feeding (Figure 3-27) and covered with a gauze square (A). This serves as a safety valve and prevents gastric reflux and abdominal distention. It may be lowered and left open to provide constant decompression (B); or it may be clamped in preparation for home care or removal (C).

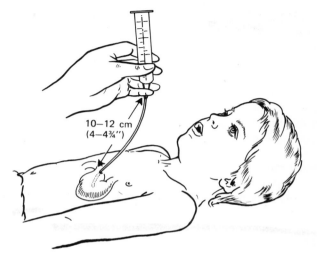

10—12 cm
(4—4¾")

Figure 3-26.

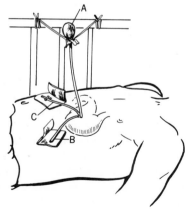

Figure 3-27.

If the tube is to be clamped, instill enough water to clear the tubing (10 to 30 milliliters, depending on length of tubing), then clamp before all of water leaves syringe. If the tube is to be left open, it is not necessary to add water.

Record procedure accurately, including type and amount of feeding, amount of residual aspirate, how child tolerated feeding, any abdominal distention, and activity after feeding.

Total Parenteral Nutrition
Total parenteral nutrition (TPN), or hyperalimentation, is a means of providing complete nutrition by the intravenous route and is used when oral or gavage feedings are insufficient or impossible. The TPN fluid contains water, protein, glucose, calories, vitamins, minerals, and electrolytes. It is administered at a constant rate via an indwelling catheter and an infusion pump. TPN may be used for several months.

The TPN fluid is prepared in the pharmacy under sterile conditions. It may be stored in the refrigerator for five days and hung at room temperature for no more than 24 hours. The fluid is hypertonic and rich in nutrients; therefore, it is an excellent culture medium for bacteria. Every precaution must be taken to avoid infection in the child because of the constant hazard of sepsis. A millipore filter is used between the infusion tubing and the Silastic catheter to filter particulate matter and/or microorganisms. Medications block the filter and are added via a T-connector between the filter and the Silastic catheter. (Controversy exists over the administration of medications via the TPN tubing because of the danger of introducing infection or an air embolus. If your institution adheres to the policy of not administering medications through the TPN tubing, administer medications via a separate IV line.)

The flow rate is calculated by the physician for maximum glucose tolerance and should not exceed 10 percent of the ordered rate per hour. Do not attempt to "catch up" TPN fluids because the high osmolality of the concentrated dextrose will cause hyperglycemia and an osmotic diuresis leading to dehydration, seizures, and coma. Sudden reduction or cessation of the flow rate will cause hypoglycemia. Monitor flow rate every hour to avoid these complications.

Central Venous Hyperalimentation
Figure 3-28 illustrates central venous hyperalimentation. A Silastic catheter is threaded from the jugular vein into the superior vena cava (A) under sterile conditions. The catheter is tunneled subcutaneously from the vein entry point in the neck (B) to a skin exit site away from the incision (C). Moving the exit site to a remote point lessens the chance of blood contamination from skin organisms. The catheter is secured with subcutaneous sutures. An antibacterial ointment and sterile dressing are applied to the exit site. A coil of catheter (F) is included in the dressing to avoid acciden-

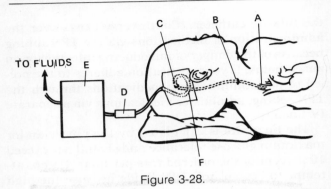

Figure 3-28.

tal displacement. Also shown in Figure 3-28 are millipore filter (D) and infusion pump (E).

Due to the location of the catheter in the vena cava, a break in the line could cause exsanguination or an air embolism precipitated by deep inspiration. A padded Kelly clamp is kept at the bedside to occlude the catheter should a break occur. All equipment is changed daily with the exception of the Silastic catheter. The dressing is changed when the equipment is changed, using strict aseptic technique. Expose the insertion site without putting any tension on the catheter itself. Examine the site for redness, swelling, or loose sutures. At least two sutures should be intact. Sediment in tubing may indicate infection, but cloudiness of the plastic tubing may be caused by the providone-iodine (Betadine) and may be mistaken for sediment. Check for kinks or small leaks in line. Clean skin with a Betadine scrub solution on a 4-inch gauze square; rinse, then dry. Apply a folded sterile 2-inch square with Betadine ointment directly over insertion site and paint the area to be taped with benzoin. Loop a coil of tubing in outer dressing (F) to prevent tension on sutures. Tape the dressing securely and reinforce as needed.

When changing infusion tubing, clamp the catheter with a padded Kelly clamp to prevent introduction of air into vena cava. Filters are cultured weekly to determine if infection is present before clinical symptoms appear. Wipe all joints in the infusion circuit with Betadine b.i.d. to remove any traces of nutrient solution and to aid in preventing infection. Antibiotics are given only if child's underlying condition warrants.

Peripheral Hyperalimentation
Peripheral hyperalimentation therapy may be more advantageous at times than central venous hyperalimentation. TPN can be offered with a 10 percent glucose concentration via peripheral infusions for short periods of time (several weeks). Nursing management and monitoring are essentially the same, although no dressing changes are needed. Careful observation of the infusion site is necessary because of the irritating properties of hyperalimentation fluids. Infiltration may cause sloughing of the skin severe enough to require skin grafts. If the IV infiltrates, remove it at once and notify physician.

Figure 3-29 shows a means of introducing fat emulsions (lipids) to supplement therapy with hypertonic dextrose solutions. Because fat is a more concentrated form of energy, it supplies more calories in a small amount of water. Fat emulsions are isotonic and thus are less hazardous than hypertonic dextrose solutions. Intralipid 10 percent is a fat emulsion made from egg yolk, soybean oil, phospholipids, and glycerin and is best given peripherally. No more than 4 gm/kg/24 hours should be administered. No drugs, other fluids, or electrolytes can be added to fat emulsions, nor can

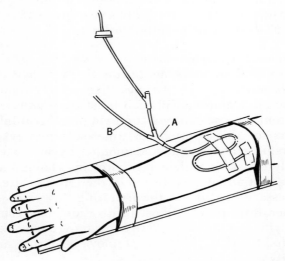

Figure 3-29.

an in-line filter be used because it breaks up the emulsion. Hypertonic dextrose solutions can be given through a separate line that connects with the fat emulsion via a Y-connector *only* at the site of infusion (A). The lipid line must be the *lower* line (B) at the Y connection, or the lipids, which are heavier than the hyperalimentation fluids, will back up into the hyperalimentation fluid. Two infusion pumps are required: one for fat emulsion and one for hypertonic dextrose solutions.

Watch for transient side effects, such as vomiting, shivering, fever, chills, flushing, and pain in the chest and back. Delayed reactions are also possible. Report any of these side effects to the physician immediately. Urine checks for sugar and acetone are done every four hours to assess the child's tolerance for glucose.

GASTRIC DECOMPRESSION

Gastric decompression may be used preoperatively to prevent vomiting and postoperatively to prevent stomach distension caused by swallowed air and gastric secretions. Maintaining a patent tube is mandatory; if the tube is blocked, vomiting and aspiration may occur.

Equipment

Salem-Sump (double lumen) tube: Size #10 French for the six- to ten-year-old; #12 to 16 French for adolescents. (These sizes are guidelines only.)

Feeding tube (single lumen) for the infant or young child
Irrigating syringe
Irrigation fluid

Procedure for Gastric Decompression

Figure 3-30 shows a Salem-Sump tube: (A)—Large lumen (drainage or main lumen). (B)—Smaller lumen (sump or air lumen) which provides continuous airflow and controls the amount of suction at gastric mucosa. (C)—Blue pigtail connects to air lumen. (D)—Single lumen feeding tube is shown for comparison. To insert tubing, measure as for gastric gavage and check for proper insertion.

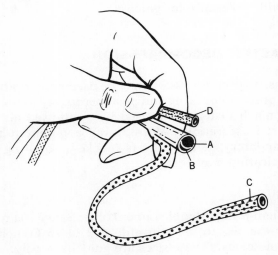

Figure 3-30.

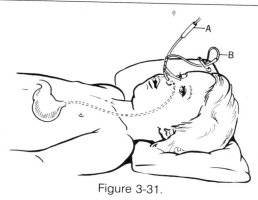

Figure 3-31.

In Figure 3-31 the tube may be connected to low suction via a 5-in-1 connector (**A**) or to gravity (straight) drainage. Gravity drainage is preferred for infants. Do not pinch or close blue pigtail (**B**) during suctioning or sump action will be eliminated. Keep pigtail above patient's midline to avoid reflux into pigtail.

Procedure for Irrigating

1. With suction source on, irrigate sump lumen with air (2 milliliters for infant, 5 to 10 milliliters for adolescents) through blue pigtail. This assures that tubing is not touching stomach mucosa.

2. Disconnect tubing from suction source and remove 5-in-1 connector. Attach irrigating syringe to main lumen and irrigate. (If physician has not ordered a specific solution, use normal saline—5 to 10 milliliters for infants and 20 milliliters for adolescents.)

3. Reconnect main lumen to suction source. To check patency of sump lumen, irrigate sump lumen again with air.
4. If feedings or medications are administered through tube, discontinue suction for 15 to 20 minutes and irrigate tubing to maintain patency.

BIBLIOGRAPHY

Bode, H.H. and Warshal, J.B. (eds): Parenteral Nutrition in infancy and childhood, in *Advances in Experimental Medicine and Biology,* vol. 46. New York, Plenum Press, 1974.

Conway, A. and Williams, T. Parenteral alimentation. *American Journal of Nursing* 76:574, 1976.

Fischer J.E. (ed): *Total Parenteral Nutrition.* Boston, Little Brown & Co., 1976.

Ghadimi, H. (ed): *Total Parenteral Nutrition Premises and Promises.* New York, John Wiley & Sons, Inc., 1975.

McConnell, E.A. Ensuring safer stomach suctioning with the Salem Sump tube. *Nursing '77* 7:54, September, 1977.

Raffensperger, J.G. and Fochtman D: Nursing care of the child with gastrointestinal anolmalies, in Fochtman D. and Raffensperger, J.G. (eds). *Principles of Nursing Care for the Pediatric Surgery Patient,* ed. 2. Boston, Little Brown & Co., 1976, p. 35.

McFarlane J.M., Whitson, B.J., Hartley, L.M. *Contemporary Pediatric Nursing : A Conceptual Approach.* New York, John Wiley & Sons, Inc., 1980.

Ziemer, M. and Carroll J.S. Infant gavage reconsidered. *American Journal of Nursing* 78:1543, 1978.

CHAPTER 4

Oxygenation Needs of the Child

OXYGEN THERAPY

Oxygen (O_2) is administered to the child via a tent, nasal catheter, mask, incubator, or hood. The administration of oxygen requires a physician's order except in an emergency. An inspired oxygen level of 30 to 100 percent is necessary for most oxygen deficits. Tents can deliver about 40 percent oxygen; nasal catheters, about 50 percent; tight-fitting masks, about 100 percent; incubators, 40 to 100 percent; and hoods, about 100 percent. Levels of over 40 percent are not administered unless ordered by the physician. Hyperoxemia (PaO_2 [partial pressure of oxygen in arterial blood] well above the normal range of 60 to 100 mmHg) may cause retrolental fibroplasia in the newborn, especially in the premature infant. However, the danger lies in a heightened *blood level* of oxygen, not in an increased fraction of inspired oxygen concentration (FIO_2). The FIO_2 may be 100 percent, and the child's PaO_2 may be only 40. Oxygen toxicity is a complication of oxygen therapy; it is suspected

117

when the PaO_2 drops in the presence of an increasing FIO_2.

Use an oxygen analyzer every two to four hours to monitor oxygen concentration. Blood gas studies may be done when the child is receiving oxygen therapy. (See Table 4-1.)

Oxygen is heated before it is administered to premature and full-term newborns. Because oxygen dries the tissues, it must be humidified before it reaches the child. Sterile water is used for this purpose, along with other agents deemed necessary by the physician, such as bronchodilators, mucolytic agents, and antibiotics. Thus, a fine mist that goes deep into the airways and helps loosen secretions is produced. The mist may soak the child's clothes and linens; change as necessary.

Safety principles are a must when oxygen is in use. Although oxygen itself will not burn, it *supports combustion*. The more oxygen present, the more readily fires start, and the faster they burn. If a spark ignites in the presence of increased oxygen, an explosive, raging fire can start. In the presence of pure oxygen, fuels can burn without the aid of a spark. All oxygen gauges are labeled "Use no oil"; this refers not only to lubricating oil but also to hair oil or lip lubricants other than water-soluble types. Volatile chemicals, such as alcohols, ether, and antiseptic tinctures, should not be used. Electrical equipment, such as portable x-ray machines, heating pads, and electrical toys are prohibited, as are wool and synthetic fibers, which generate static electricity. Stuffed toys that retain moisture (and

Table 4-1. Normal and Abnormal Blood Gas Measurements

	pH	P_{CO_2}	HCO_3^- (mEq/liter)	CO_2
Normal values				
Child	7.35–7.45	35–45	24–26	25–28
Term Infant:				
birth	7.26–7.29	54.5		
1 hr	7.30	38.8		20.6
3 hr	7.34	38.3		21.9
1 to 3 days	7.38–7.41	34–35		21.4
Premature				
>1250 gm:				
1 to 3 days	7.38–7.39	38–39		
<1250 gm:				
1 to 3 days	7.35–7.36	37–44		
Abnormal values				
Metabolic acidosis	↓	↓	↓	↓
Acute respiratory acidosis	↓	↑	⟷	Sl. ↑
Compensated respiratory acidosis	⟷ or Sl. ↓	↑	↑	↑
Metabolic alkalosis	↑	Sl. ↑	↑	↑
Acute respiratory alkalosis	↑	↓	⟷	Sl. ↓
Compensated respiratory alkalosis	⟷ or Sl. ↑	↓	↓	↓

therefore, bacteria) also are not permitted. "No Smoking" signs must be posted when oxygen is used.

Oxygen therapy is terminated gradually. Unzip the tent or raise the canopy over support rods; open air vents in incubator (but do this with caution, because infants have fallen through open air vents); or decrease the liter flow for hoods. Monitor the child's respiratory status frequently. Watch for restlessness, tachycardia, tachypnea, and cyanosis. If the child experiences any respiratory difficulty, return oxygen therapy to original status and notify physician.

Oxygen Analyzer

Oxygen concentration (in tents, hoods, incubators, etc.) is measured with an oxygen analyzer. Analyzers are calibrated to measure 100 percent in pure oxygen in the respiratory therapy department before being used on the unit.

An oxygen analyzer is illustrated in Figure 4-1. To check oxygen concentration, test the battery by pressing battery check button (A); the needle should register in green area (between 80 and 100) if battery is charged (B). Turn the on-off switch (C) to 100; if the needle does not register at 21 percent in room air, turn the balance knob (D) to set needle at 21 percent. Remove probe (E) and place it inside tent, hood, and so on. The needle will move to register concentration of oxygen. Turn the analyzer off, replace the probe, and record oxygen concentration.

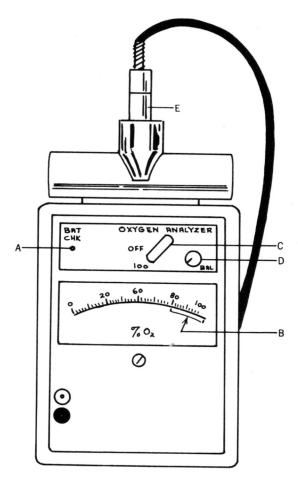

Figure 4-1.

121

Infant Oxygen Hood

The oxygen hood is a clear, sturdy dome that fits over the infant's head to provide a high concentration of oxygen. It may be used in an incubator, radiant warmer, or open crib. Various brands and sizes are available to fit the infant weighing 1 to 8 kilograms (2 to 18 pounds). Carbon dioxide escapes through the neck opening; this also serves as a safety feature should the oxygen system fail.

Equipment

Hood
Oxygen analyzer with probe
Sterile water
Thermometer (included with hood)
Corrugated tubing
Nebulizer or humidifier
Heating probe
Flow regulator

Procedure for the Infant Oxygen Hood

Figure 4-2 illustrates the Shiley Infant Oxygen Hood. Plug the flow regulator into the wall and attach the nebulizer/humidifier. Place the heating probe into nebulizer/humidifier and plug into wall outlet. Fill the nebulizer/humidifier with sterile water.

Connect the corrugated inlet tubing (A) to oxygen source and nebulizer/humidifier; attach other end to hood. Check tubing frequently for water accumulation. Unhook one end of tubing and drain water

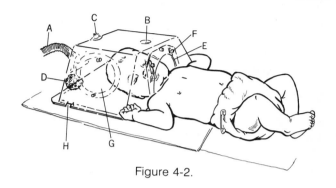

Figure 4-2.

into a basin as necessary.

Insert oxygen analyzer probe through port at top of hood (**B**). Turn oxygen source to desired level. Check concentration several times during the first hour and each time neck opening is adjusted or other changes made.

Place thermometer in port at back of hood (**C**).

Place sound baffle and water collection pad (**D**) in hood below thermometer port to reduce noise level and soak up excess moisture. Change pad when saturated. Make sure that an adequate amount of warm, moist oxygen is flowing into hood. Check temperature in hood.

Slide neck plate (**E**) to maximum opening and place infant under hood.

Adjust neck plate using the thumbscrews on slide (**F**). Leave space between the infant and the neck plate for escape of carbon dioxide; this space also serves as a safety device should the oxygen source fail.

There are side entry panels (G) on either side for easy access to infant's head. Check oxygen concentration with panels closed. There is an inlet (H) on either side for two IV lines.

Tents

A variety of oxygen tents for the child are available. Each carries with it instructions for use. The principles are the same, however, regardless of the brand.

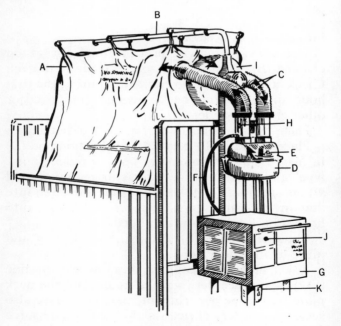

Figure 4-3.

Procedure for Oxygen Tents

The OHIO ® Pediatric Aerosol Tent shown in Figure 4-3 is designed to provide a water-saturated atmosphere for cooling. Mist is provided by a nebulizer that uses either oxygen or compressed air as a power source.

Canopy (A) is held by a canopy support rod (B). *After* air or oxygen flow is started and tent is cool, place the child in tent and tuck canopy under mattress around patient. If flow is not at least 10 liters per minute (l.p.m.), excess carbon dioxide may build up in tent.

Supply and return hoses (C) connect nebulizer to canopy and serve as a recirculating reservoir (see arrows).

Pneumatic nebulizer (D), filled either with 2500 milliliters water for eight-hour operation or a prescribed amount of medication, which is added through inlet chimney (E).

Air or oxygen source (F).

"No Smoking" signs should be posted on the door and inside the patient's room. (Note "No Smoking" sign on canopy.)

Refrigeration compressor for cooling (G).

Damper valve adjustment (H); controls damper valve and may be set at full open to permit maximum recirculation of air.

Fan to circulate air surrounding the patient (I).

"Off," "Cool," or "Circulate" selector (J). "Cool" mode will provide cooling within two minutes. "Circulate" mode will not cool, but fan will circulate air inside canopy and is used when cooling is not desired.

Condensate bottle (K) to trap moisture that collects during cooling.

Infant Incubator

Incubators provide the neonate ˙with a stable environmental temperature, isolation from infection, and oxygen as well as humidification.

The ISOLETTE® infant incubator by Air-Shields, Inc. is depicted in Figure 4-4. When the unit is plugged into power source, either Air Temperature Control lamp (T) or Skin Temperature Control lamp (N) will light, indicating that power is on and that air circulation system is operating. The various parts of the ISOLETTE are:

Clear plastic hood for easy visualization of infant (A).

Front access panel that can be lowered to horizontal position to provide a base for sliding mattress platform (B).

Arm ports for sterile access to infant (C).

Elbow latch to open arm ports (D). Use gentle pressure with elbows to release latch.

Knobs to release front access panel (E).

Mattress and sliding mattress platform (F). Lower front access panel, then slide mattress platform out.

Mattress elevators (G). Turn to elevate end of mattress to place infant in Fowler or Trendelenburg positions. When mattress is not elevated, levers should point toward ends of ISOLETTE ®.

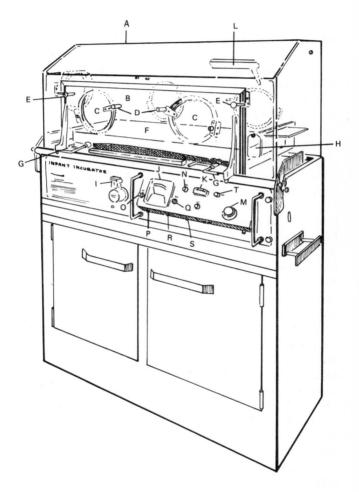

Figure 4-4.

Access holes for easy access to IV tubing (H), and so on, covered with pivoting plate when not in use.

Humidity chamber (I). Fill chamber with distilled sterile water. Single filling will last one full day on maximum humidity setting. Turn fill chamber to left to drain humidity reservoir. It should be drained completely and refilled daily. Set Humidity Control Knob at left end of hood (not shown) to desired level.

Infant Servo Control (ISC) display meter (J). Patient probe attaches to infant's abdomen and his abdominal skin temperature, which correlates to his body temperature, is displayed on control panel. Heater output is controlled to keep infant's body temperature at desired control point. Normally, air temperature within the ISOLETTE ® does not exceed 37.2°C (99°F). Should this system fail, an alarm will sound, the heater will shut off, and a safety thermostat will operate at 37.8° to 39.4°C (100° to 103°F).

Heater Output Meter (K) provides continuous indication of heat required to maintain a given skin temperature. Changes in heater output, which correlate with changes in the infant's heat requirements, serve as a diagnostic tool for assessing physiologic and metabolic alterations in the infant. These changes provide an indication of the infant's dependency on his environmental temperature for maintenance of his own body temperature.

Hood thermometer (L) indicates temperature inside incubator.

To Maintain Skin Temperature Control

1. Turn Air Temperature Control knob (M) clockwise to click position (skin temperature control) so that Skin Temperature control lamp (N) is lighted. Rotating clockwise without clicking sets ISOLETTE ® for maximum heat with control maintained by air temperature rather than skin temperature. The danger of accidentally overheating the infant thus is present.

2. Check calibration periodically by pressing the Red Line Adjust button (O). The meter needle should align itself with the red line on ISC meter face (J). If it doesn't, keep button depressed and turn red line adjust screw (P) until needle stops on red line. Tap the meter face gently to stabilize needle.

3. To set skin temperature prescribed by physician, press Control Point Adjust button (Q) and, when needle stops, turn Control Point Adjust screw (R) until the needle stops at desired temperature control point.

4. Insert the plug of Patient Probe into socket (S). Clean the infant's abdomen, and cover the probe with a piece of cotton (to minimize effects of air temperature on probe); then tape probe halfway between xiphoid process and umbilicus, or in the axilla. The ISC will provide a continuous indication of the infant's skin temperature.

To Maintain Air Temperature Control

1. Turn Air Temperature Control knob (M) coun-

terclockwise until Air Temperature Control lamp (T) is lighted. Check hood thermometer (L) for ISOLETTE ® temperature (usually reached within one hour). When the prescribed temperature is indicated, rotate Air Temperature Control knob counterclockwise until the Heater Output Meter (K) indicates "½." The temperature within the unit will now be automatically maintained within 0.5°C (1°F) of the prescribed temperature read on hood thermometer. To raise or lower incubator temperature, turn Air Temperature Control knob to right or left. When Air Temperature Control is in use, the infant's skin temperature can be *monitored* on the ISC meter. *This mode will not control heater output*.

Oxygen Administration

Connect tubing from oxygen source to oxygen inlet valve on back of ISOLETTE. Adjust oxygen flow to deliver desired concentration according to chart on back of ISOLETTE (and below). An oxygen limiter prevents a high concentration of oxygen from flowing into the ISOLETTE. With the red flag on back of ISOLETTE in the *down*, or horizontal, position, oxygen concentration is limited to 40 percent. If, however, the infant requires a higher concentration to raise his oxygen tension to normal levels, up to 90 percent concentration may be administered by raising the red flag to the up position. This reduces the air intake; thus, the oxygen concentration will be higher. The red flag serves as a reminder that a higher concentration of oxygen is being administered. If the oxygen flow is accidently terminated with the flag in the up position, the emergency air intake port will allow 6 to 8 lpm flow of room air into the isolette.

Flow of Oxygen liter/minute (lpm)	Concentration of Oxygen
Flag Down Position	
4	27−30%
6	30−35%
8	35−40%
Flag Up Position	
8	65%*
10	70%
12	75%

*These are minimum concentration percentages of oxygen.

TRACHEOSTOMY CARE

A tracheostomy is usually performed to bypass an upper airway obstruction or to provide long-term intubation; for example, for burns of the respiratory tract. Tubes are usually made of polyvinyl chloride (PVC) or silicone, rather than metal. These tubes are lightweight, soft, and pliable and therefore conform more comfortably to the contour of the trachea. Some are radiopaque, permitting visualization of the insertion position with x-ray films.

Most pediatric tubes do not have an inner cannula because the smooth plastic surface reduces crust formation. Plastic tubes are changed approximately once a week. Pediatric tracheostomy tubes are usually not cuffed; rather, an appropriate-size tube is chosen to fit the trachea. The size of the child's trachea is roughly equal to that of his little finger.

Since a tracheostomy bypasses the body's normal filtering, warming, and humidifying systems in the upper airway, air must be warmed and humidified by artificial means to prevent drying and to help loosen secretions. A mist tent, humidifier, nebulizer, or T-tube may be used to moisten and warm the inspired air. Continuous ultrasonic nebulization is never used for the infant, and rarely for the older child, because it delivers a high volume of water, which can cause water intoxication.

The tube is not disturbed, even to change the ties, for 72 hours after surgery because the tracheostomy tract is not well-formed until this time, and the danger of displacement is great. Have the following emergency equipment at the bedside: extra sterile tracheostomy tube and obturator, endotracheal intubation kit, AMBU bag with adapter to fit tracheostomy tube, and sterile hemostat taped to the head of the bed (to hold open the stoma should the tube become displaced). The infant or small child will have to be restrained to keep him from pulling his tracheostomy tube out. Be sure his toys are too big to be pushed down the tube. Observe him carefully so that he does not occlude the tube with toys, clothes, blankets, and so on.

Procedure for a Tracheostomy

Figure 4-5 illustrates a Shiley disposable pediatric tracheostomy tube (A) with obturator (B), which is available in infant's and children's sizes. It is radiopaque for x-ray determination of proper positioning.

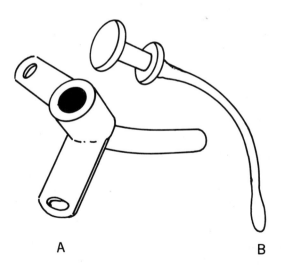

A   B

Figure 4-5.

Size	Outer Diameter	Inner Diameter	Length	Suction Catheter Size
00	4.5 mm (#14 French)	3.1 mm	39 mm	#8 French
0	5.0 mm (#15 French)	3.4 mm	40 mm	#10 French
1	5.5 mm (#17 French)	3.7 mm	41 mm	#12 French
2	6.0 mm (#18 French)	4.1 mm	42 mm	#14 French
3	7.0 mm (#21 French)	4.8 mm	44 mm	#16 French
4	8.0 mm (#24 French)	5.5 mm	46 mm	#18 French

Never leave the infant or young child with a tracheostomy alone (Figure 4-6). The child is frightened because he cannot make a sound; he cannot even hear himself cry. The child has no way to communicate with you verbally; therefore, you must position yourself so that you can see him at all times. Take his vital signs at regular intervals. A fast pulse and restlessness are early signs of oxygen deprivation. The properly placed tracheostomy tube prevents any type of vocal sound; therefore, any sign of an attempt to vocalize must be interpreted as a cry for help. After the initial period of adjustment the older child may be left for short periods, provided he can use the call bell (which should be placed within easy reach). Give the child a "magic slate" or pad and pen so that he can write notes to you.

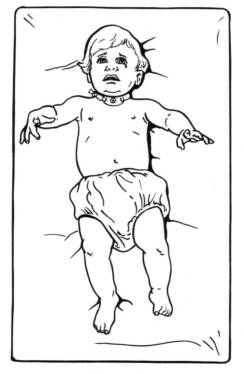

Figure 4-6.

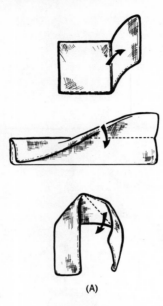

(A)

Figure 4-7A.

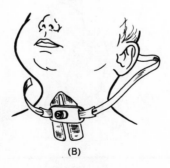

(B)

Figure 4-7B.

Observe stoma site for bleeding, crusts, irritation, and broken skin. Clean the site every four
hours with a cotton-tipped applicator moistened
with warm water. Dry carefully. To change sponge,
refold a sterile two-inch gauze square as shown in
Figure 4-7a; then insert around stoma, under
tracheostomy tube, Figure 4-7b. This technique
eliminates the necessity of cutting a gauze square
with resultant frayed ends which may be aspirated.

Two people are required to change tracheostomy
ties (Figure 4-8). Use twill tape or commercially
prepared ties with a slit cut ½ inch from the end. If
twill tape is used, slit the hole with a hemostat
(scissors will cut the fibers, fraying the tie and
perhaps pulling it apart). Remove old ties and have

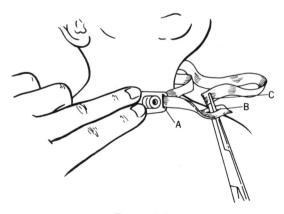

Figure 4-8.

assistant hold tube securely in place while you replace ties. Thread end of tape up through flange slit
(A), using hemostat to pull it through. Then, insert
hemostat through slit in tie (B), grasp other end of
tie (C), and pull it through the hole. Pull firmly
until the tie locks securely at flange. Repeat for
other side.

With assistant flexing child's neck with one hand
and securing tube with the other, bring tie around
and behind to the opposite side of neck and tie in a
square knot at side of neck (Figure 4-9). Flexing the
neck reduces its circumference, thus loosening the
tie. If tape is tied with neck extended, it may loosen
and permit the tube to become dislodged when the
child flexes his neck and coughs.

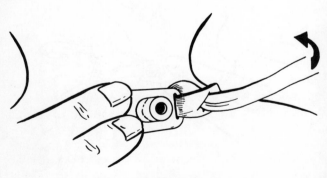

Figure 4-9.

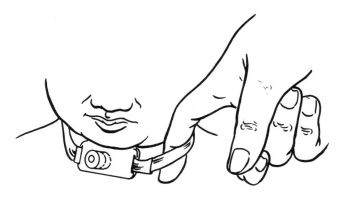

Figure 4-10.

Test tie for tension by placing one finger between tape and neck with child's neck flexed (Figure 4-10). Because the infant has extra skin folds under his chin, he may become restless and cough when his flexed neck occludes his tracheostomy tube. Explain this to the parents before you check the tie tension so they know that coughing is to be expected, and that testing the tie tension is necessary.

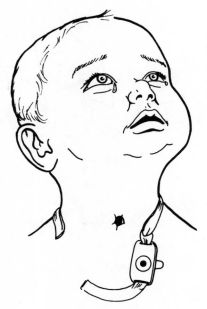

Figure 4-11.

If the tube is not tied securely around the neck, it is easily displaced, causing possible respiratory distress and death within minutes (Figure 4-11).

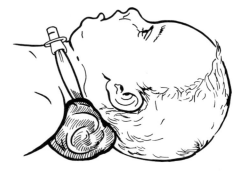

Figure 4-12.

Because the infant has a short neck, his chin may occlude the tracheostomy tube (Figure 4-12). For this reason, his head must be extended at all times. A sponge-rubber wedge or rolled towel is used to extend the head. Be sure clothes do not cover the tube opening. Do not tie any clothes, such as night shirts, around the neck; keep bed linens below the nipple line.

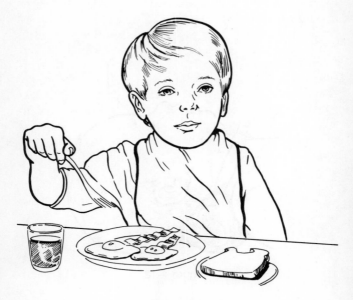

Figure 4-13.

When the infant eats, cover the tube with a moistened gauze sponge to prevent aspiration of food into the trachea. The older child may use a bib with short ties as shown (Figure 4-13).

Suctioning

Tracheostomy suctioning requires sterile technique to avoid introducing bacteria into the trachea and bronchi. Select the proper catheter size relative to the lumen of the tracheostomy tube. (See the chart presented earlier for a guide to catheter size.) Using a too-large catheter will cause aspiration of oxygen from the airways, resulting in hypoxia. Vagal stimulation is also a possibility, and may result in cardiac arrest. Assisted ventilation with a manual respirator (AMBU bag) is usually ordered for three to five minutes before suctioning. Suction as ordered or as necessary (from every ten minutes to every two hours).

Equipment

Sterile gloves
Sterile catheter
Sterile syringe
Sterile bowl
Sterile 0.9 percent normal saline

Procedure for Suctioning

Figure 4-14 illustrates the suctioning procedure. Wash hands. Open sterile gloves, catheter, syringe, saline, and bowl. Pour a small amount of saline into bowl. Don sterile gloves; draw 2.0 milliliter's of saline into syringe. Place syringe on sterile field, and remove catheter from wrapping; fold tip of catheter into palm of gloved hand. With the other hand, insert 0.5 to 2.0 milliliters of saline into trachea to loosen secretions. Quickly attach the tubing from suction machine to catheter (with hand to be contaminated). Moisten the catheter with sterile saline. (Note: After saline is introduced into trachea, the child may begin to cough and gag; therefore, you must move quickly to suction him. This procedure may require two people: one to insert saline into trachea and one to suction immediately.) In some institutions it is routine for two people to suction the tracheostomy.

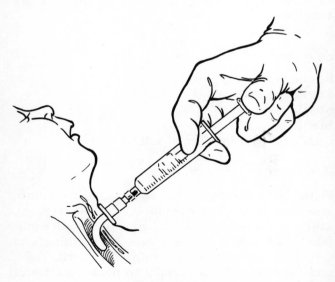

Figure 4-14.

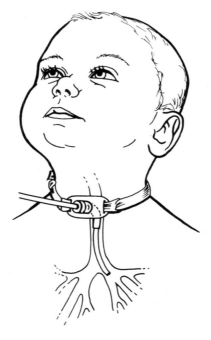

Figure 4-15.

With contaminated hand, turn the child's head
to right side to suction left bronchus (Figure 4-15).

With suction off, insert catheter into tube until the child coughs (Figure 4-16).

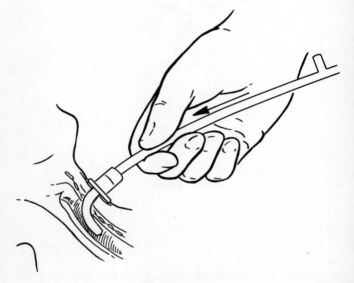

Figure 4-16.

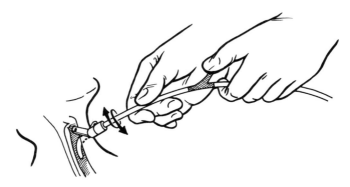

Figure 4-17.

Advance catheter to main stem bronchus during inspiration following cough (Figure 4-17). Using continuous rotating motion, withdraw catheter quickly as you apply intermittent suction by occluding and releasing suction valve ("T" or "Y" opening). This step should take less than 15 seconds. During the first 24 hours after tracheostomy, use a new sterile catheter each time you enter trachea. Otherwise, let the child rest a few minutes and breathe humidified oxygen after each suction episode. Repeat suctioning as necessary to clear airway.

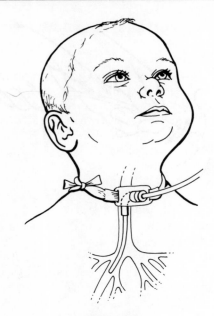

Figure 4-18.

To suction right bronchus, turn the child's head to left (Figure 4-18). Discard catheter and gloves. Check the ties and cleanse around stoma as necessary. Check the child's vital signs and be sure he is comfortable. Observe for respiratory distress. Record procedure, how the child tolerated it, character of secretions, and any respiratory distress. Let the child rest.

CARDIOPULMONARY RESUSCITATION

Cardiopulmonary resuscitation (CPR) is a rapid sequence of actions performed as emergency measures to restore ventilation and circulation. The child may suffer irreversible brain damage in three to five minutes after breathing and circulation stop. Your actions are critical to his survival. If CPR is effective, the child's color will improve and his pupils will constrict to normal size. CPR is never interrupted for more than five seconds for any reason; it is continued until spontaneous respirations and a palpable pulse return, or until a physician determines that the child is not responding and pronounces him dead.

Medications, such as epinephrine, sodium bicarbonate, isoproterenol, and calcium chloride, may be given to stimulate cardiopulmonary function. If ventricular arrhythmias are present, direct-current defibrillation is used to deliver asynchronized shock to the chest in an effort to interrupt the fibrillation. After successful resuscitation, the child is placed in an intensive care setting until he is no longer at risk.

To give CPR effectively, you need special training by a CPR instructor. The procedure presented here will serve as a review for your CPR training. Remember the ABC's of CPR: *a*irway; *b*reathing; *c*irculation.

Procedure for CPR

Establish Unresponsiveness: If infant appears to be

unconscious, shake him and shout in his ear, "Baby, Baby, are you all right?" Flick his toes. Turn him on his back. *Call for help.* Allow three to five seconds to establish unresponsiveness; be sure child is not just sleeping soundly.

Airway (Figure 4-19): Tip infant's head back to open the airway and check for breathlessness. Hyperextend neck of older child and pull his jaw forward and up. Do not hyperextend infant's neck (it will narrow his airway). Place your ear over his mouth, *look* at his chest, *listen* for breath sounds, and *feel* for air movement. Child may begin to breathe after his airway is opened. Allow three to five seconds to establish breathlessness.

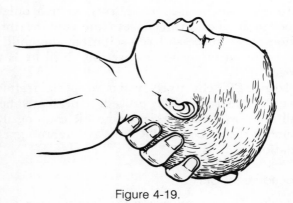

Figure 4-19.

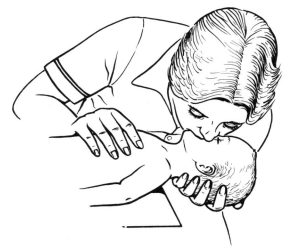

Figure 4-20.

Breathing (Figure 4-20): If infant does not start breathing, cover his mouth and nose with your mouth, forming a tight seal, and give four rapid puffs of air to oxygenate lungs. Use puffs of air from your cheeks only, to avoid over-inflating his lungs. For the older child, pinch his nose and cover only his mouth with your mouth. Inflate his chest until it begins to rise. Allow three to five seconds for these rapid ventilations.

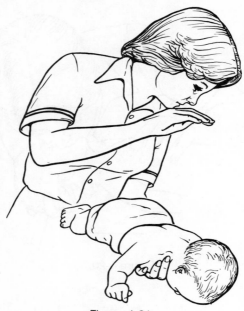

Figure 4-21.

If there is resistance to your ventilations, reposition head to be sure tongue is not obstructing airway, and repeat four rapid ventilations.

If there is continued resistance to your ventilations, suspect complete airway blockage by a foreign body. Place infant's head down on your forearm, supporting his head with your hand (Figure 4-21). Cup your hand and deliver four sharp, rapid blows over the spine between the shoulder blades. Be forceful; you are trying to dislodge a foreign object.

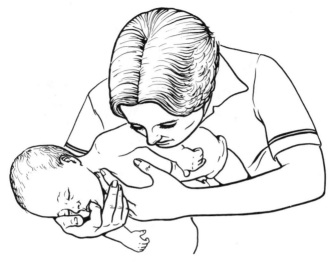

Figure 4-22.

Sweep out mouth with hooked finger (Figure 4-22). Begin inside top cheek, moving deeply into back of throat; draw out any foreign body to lower cheek, grasp and remove it. Be careful not to force the object deeper into the throat or to obstruct the airway with your finger.

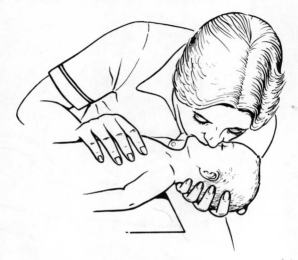

Figure 4-23.

Turn infant over and give four rapid puffs of air
(Figure 4-23). Do this whether or not you have dislodged the foreign body. Take three to five seconds
to ventilate. If airway resistance is still present and
no air seems to be entering lungs, repeat back slaps
and finger probe (Figures 4-21 and 4-22).

Gastric distension may also reduce lung volume
by elevating the diaphragm. If there is marked distension, turn infant's head to side to prevent aspiration, and use one hand to exert pressure over
epigastrium between umbilicus and rib cage.

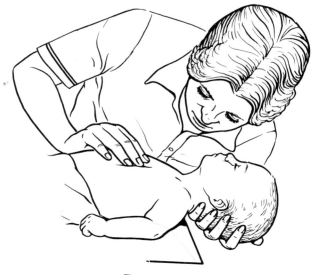

Figure 4-24.

Circulation (Figure 4-24): After you have oxygenated the lungs, check for a pulse. In infants, check apical pulse near left nipple, using the flat of your fingers. Spend five to ten seconds looking for the pulse. Count the seconds to be sure you spend sufficient time. Performing external cardiac massage on a beating heart can cause the heart to stop, so be sure there is no pulse before proceeding.

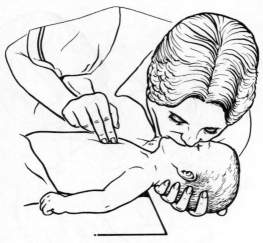

Figure 4-25.

After lack of a pulse is established, start external cardiac compressions (Figure 4-25). Place tips of index and middle finger over *midsternum* and compress 1.3 to 1.8 centimeters (½ to ¾ inch) at the rate of 80 to 100/min. Do not place fingers over lower sternum as with adults; the ventricles of the heart are higher in the chest in infants and children, and because of the pliability of the child's chest, the danger of lacerating the liver is greater.

Give one ventilation on the *upstroke* of each fifth compression. Cover nose and mouth as shown in Figure 4-23, and give a puff of air to ventilate the lungs. Leave your mouth in this position through-out resuscitation. Count out loud: one-two-three-four-five (puff), one-two-three-four-five (puff), and so on. These ventilations and compressions should be performed smoothly, and a 1:5 ratio of ventila-tions to compressions should be maintained. Be sure to ventilate on the upstroke, otherwise air cannot fully inflate the lungs.

Two-person CPR on infant, showing ventilation with a hand respirator AMBU bag is shown in Fig-ure 4-26. Note that the nurse's fingers elevate the infant's jaw to extend his neck.

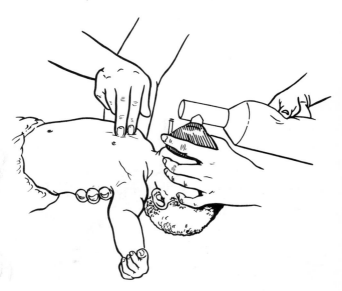

Figure 4-26.

For the young child, use the heel of one hand to compress the lower third of the sternum 1.8 to 3.8 centimeters (¾ to 1½ inch) at a rate of 80 to 100/min (Figure 4-27).

For the older child, use both hands to compress the lower third of the sternum 2.5 to 5.0 centimeters (1 to 2 inches) at a rate of 80/min (Figure 4-28).

After CPR, give care to the child as required, determine if family members are being cared for, record all events, and restock emergency cart.

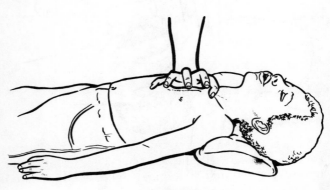

Figure 4-27.

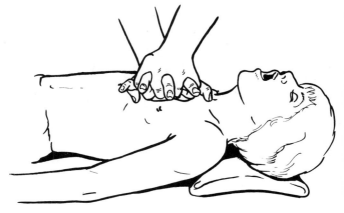

Figure 4-28.

CLEARING THE AIRWAY

Bulb Suction

A bulb syringe is often used for oral and nasal suction on infants and children when secretions are not severe enough to require more sophisticated suction techniques.

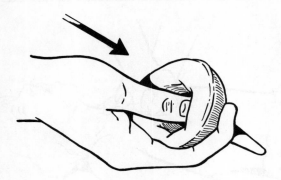

Figure 4-29.

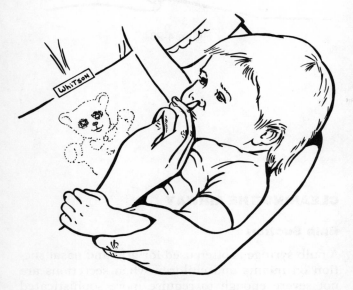

Figure 4-30.

Procedure for Bulb Suction

To suction with a bulb syringe, push bulb in with your thumb (Figure 4-29).

Holding thumb in, insert tip of syringe into the child's nose or mouth (Figure 4-30). Note that the child is held "in arms" with his right arm tucked behind nurse's back. The child's left arm is held in nurse's left hand, or vice versa if nurse is left-handed.

Release thumb providing suction (Figure 4-31).

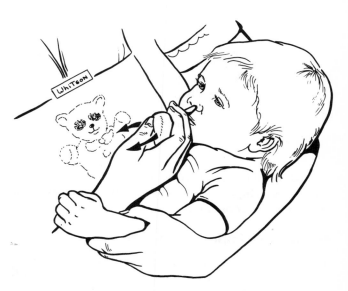

Figure 4-31.

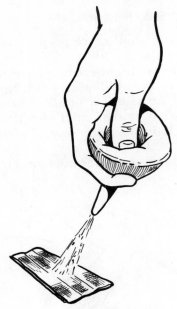

Figure 4-32.

Push bulb in again with thumb to expel contents onto tissue (Figure 4-32). Discard tissue; rinse bulb syringe with cool water.

Modified Heimlich Maneuver

This procedure is used to dislodge a foreign object, usually food, from the airway. The victim will suddenly be unable to speak and may clutch his throat in obvious distress (the universal sign of choking). He may appear cyanotic and struggle to breathe. Prompt action is necessary.

Procedure for Aiding Choking Victim

Identify complete airway obstruction by asking victim, "Can you speak?" (Figure 4-33). If he can speak, cough forcefully, and breathe adequately, do not interfere with his efforts to expel the foreign object. If victim is a child or infant, do not place him head-down if he can breathe adequately in the upright position. Suspect complete airway obstruc-

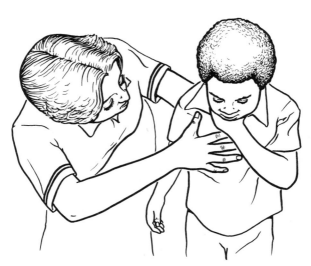

Figure 4-33.

tion if victim cannot speak, has a weak cough, and makes high-pitched crowing sounds when trying to breathe. Tell victim you are going to help him.

If the airway is completely obstructed, bend the child forward slightly and use the heel of your hand to deliver four sharp blows rapidly and forcefully to the spine between the shoulder blades. Support child's chest with your other arm while delivering blows to back.

To deliver manual thrusts, find correct landmarks before delivering abdominal or chest thrusts (Figure 4-34). Stand behind the child and wrap

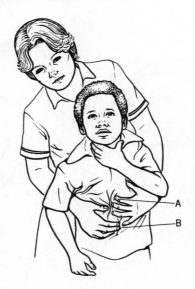

Figure 4-34.

your arms around his waist; locate xiphoid process
(A) with one of your hands and the umbilicus (B)
with the other.

Place fist, thumb side in, at the point midway
between xiphoid process and umbilicus (Figure
4-35). Thrusting higher than this point may be inef-
fective and waste precious time.

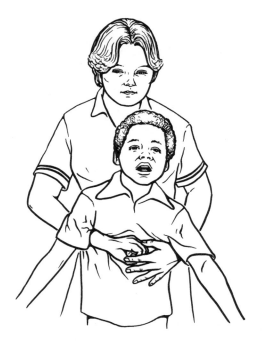

Figure 4-35.

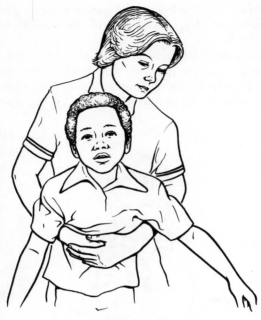

Figure 4-36.

With fist in position, grasp it with your other hand and thrust in and up forcefully four times (Figure 4-36). *Look* at the victim to see if he is still having difficulty breathing. If so, repeat four back blows and four abdominal thrusts until airway is clear.

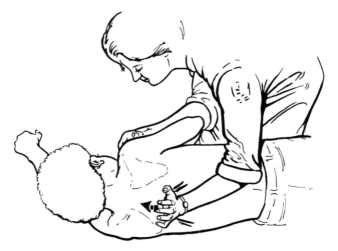

Figure 4-37.

Chest thrusts are used for the obese or pregnant person. Wrap your arms around victim's chest, under his armpits. Thrust with your fist on sternum but not over xiphoid process.

If the child is lying down and is unconscious, kneel and roll him on his side, facing you, supporting his chest with your thigh (Figure 4-37). Deliver four sharp blows with heel of your hand to the child's spine between his shoulder blades.

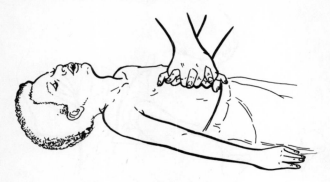

Figure 4-38.

Turn the child on his back and open his airway to deliver manual thrusts (Figure 4-38). Your knees should be close to his hips and your shoulder directly above his abdomen. Place the heel of one hand against abdomen between xiphoid process and umbilicus; place the other hand on top and press into abdomen, delivering four sharp upward thrusts.

For chest thrusts, place hands in same position as for external cardiac massage and give four rapid thrusts.

If a foreign body is at or above the level of the epiglottis, try to remove it with your fingers (Figure 4-39). Turn the child's head to side away from you and open his mouth using the crossed-finger technique, as shown. Run your index finger down inside of cheek to base of tongue and deep into throat. Hook your finger to dislodge foreign body and bring it to mouth; remove it. Do this with caution

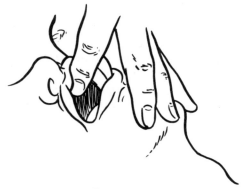

Figure 4-39.

because your finger can occlude the child's airway, and there is a danger of pushing the foreign object further into the airway.

Postural Drainage

Postural drainage is a means of positioning the patient to enhance gravity drainage of the small bronchial airways toward the trachea where secretions can be suctioned out or coughed up. Postural drainage may be done several times a day for chronic lung conditions, such as cystic fibrosis. It is most effective at bedtime (to clear secretions accumulated during the day and to promote restful sleep) and in the morning (to clear secretions accumulated during the night). Some children may need to have this procedure done every two hours or as often as five minutes of every hour.

The lung segment to be drained is placed in the uppermost position with its corresponding bronchus in as close to a vertical position as possible. Chest percussion and vibration are used with postural drainage to help dislodge secretions.

To percuss, use an appropriate instrument (Figure 4-40) or your tightly cupped hand to trap air between hand and chest. The more air trapped, the more effective the percussion. Relax your wrist and tap the chest rapidly for one full minute in each position. Correct percussion produces a hollow sound; incorrect percussion produces a slapping sound and a reddened area on the skin.

Vibration is a rapid movement made with the percussion object only during exhalation. It is done following percussion. Ask the child to take a deep

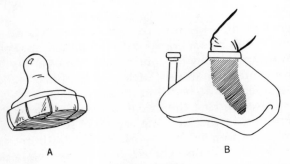

A   B

Figure 4-40.

breath; as he exhales, vibrate over percussion site for three to five exhalations. Ask the child to cough after vibration. Permit him to rest for a few minutes, then repeat until no more mucus is produced. Total treatment time is usually 15 to 30 minutes.

Never use postural drainage within one hour of a meal because vomiting may occur. If the child's condition warrants, stop the procedure. Assess respiratory status before and after procedure to evaluate success of therapy. Provide emesis basin and tissues. After procedure, assist the child to gradually assume sitting position and offer oral hygiene. Illustrations show infant percussion; the older child is placed on a bed or tilt board.

Equipment

Percussion object
Pillow
Suction apparatus (bulb syringe or wall suction)
Emesis basin and tissues

Procedure for Postural Drainage

Select a percussion object according to the child's size. It should be small enough to localize percussion to a specific lobe or segment of the child's lung. The following objects may be used: your cupped hand; a disposable nipple with rim padded with tape (Figure 4-40a); an anesthesia mask with hole taped (or simply stick your index finger through the hole to seal it) (Figure 4-40b); or a plastic medicine cup padded with tape.

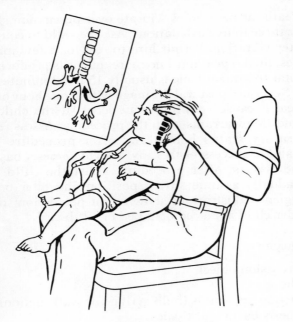

Figure 4-41.

For drainage of upper lobes, apical segments (Figure 4-41) place the child supported by a pillow, in your lap. Tilt him back against your chest. Clap above clavicle, one side at a time.

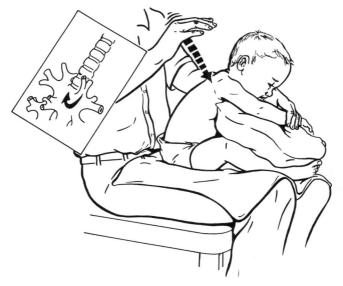

Figure 4-42.

Drainage of upper lobes, posterior segments is illustrated in Figure 4-42. Lean the child forward over a pillow in your lap. Percuss shoulders and upper back on both sides.

To drain upper lobes, anterior segments, place the child supine on a pillow in your lap (Figure 4-43). Percuss both sides of the chest between clavicle and nipple. Do not percuss over clavicle.

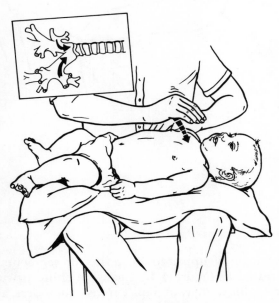

Figure 4-43.

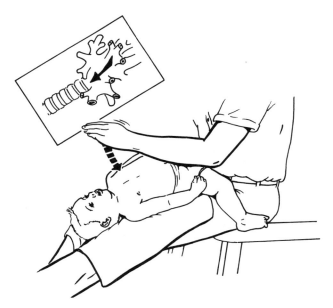

Figure 4-44.

For right middle lobe and left lingula drainage, with your legs out straight (Figure 4-44), place the child head down in your lap. To drain left lingula, turn him one-quarter turn to the right and maintain position by placing a pillow under his left side from shoulder to hip. Percuss over left nipple. Reverse to drain right middle lobe.

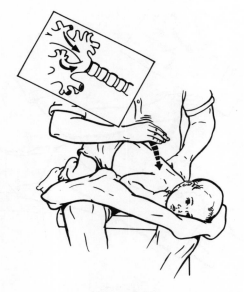

Figure 4-45.

For drainage of lower lobes, apical segments, place the child prone on a pillow on your lap or elevate his hips slightly with pillow (Figure 4-45). Percuss just below scapula on both sides.

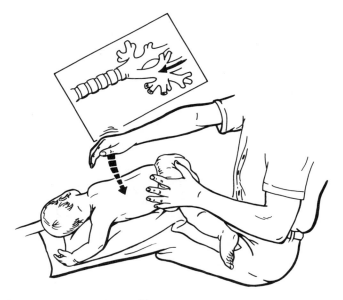

Figure 4-46.

To drain lower lobes, posterior segments, place the child prone, head down on a pillow over your extended legs (Figure 4-46). Percuss over lower ribs. Do not percuss over spine or kidneys.

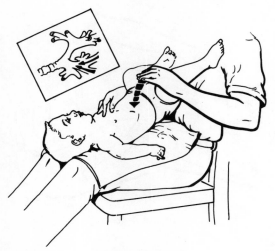

Figure 4-47.

For drainage of lower lobes, anterior segments, place the child on his back, head down on a pillow over your extended legs (Figure 4-47). Percuss over lower ribs.

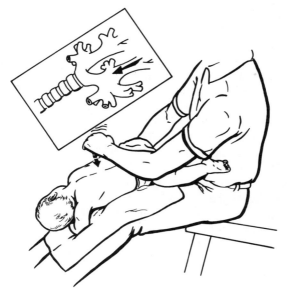

Figure 4-48.

To drain lower lobes, lateral segments see Figure 4-48. Place the child on his abdomen, head down over your extended legs. Prop him slightly on his left side with pillow, and percuss over right lower ribs to drain right side. Reverse for left side.

BIBLIOGRAPHY

Brunner, L.S. and Suddarth, D.S. *The Lippincott Manual of Nursing Practice* ed. 2. Philadelphia, J. B. Lippincott Co., 1978, p. 228–231.

Crocker, D. Management of Tracheostomy in Smith, C.A. (ed) *The Critically Ill Child Diagnosis and Management.* Philadelphia, W. B. Saunders Co., 1972, p. 139.

Hart, R. A Review of CPR for Adults. *Nursing '79* 4:54, February 1979.

Heimlich, H.J. A Life-Saving Maneuver to Prevent Food Choking. *Journal of American Medical Assn.* 234:398–401, 1975.

Kaler, J. and Kaler, H. Michael Had a Tracheostomy. *American Journal of Nursing* 74:852, 1974.

LeFort, S. Cardiopulmonary Resuscitation (CPR) Step By Step. *Canadian Nurse* 74:38, 1978.

O'Dell, A.J. The Administration of Airway Humidification. *Nursing '74* 4:67, 1974.

O'Donnell, B. and Gilmore, B.B. How to Change Tracheostomy Ties—Easily and Safely. *Nursing '78* 8:66, March 1978.

Tecklin, J.S. Positioning, Percussing, and Vibrating Patients for Effective Bronchial Drainage. *Nursing '79* 9:64, March 1979.

CHAPTER 5

Mobility Needs of the Child

HANDLING THE INFANT

Carrying the Infant

Football carry (Figure 5-1): The infant's hip rests on your hip. His head is supported with your hand; his

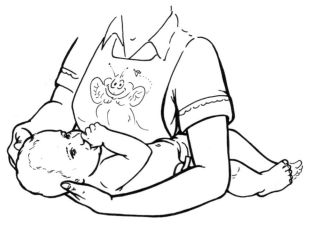

Figure 5-1.

back is supported with your forearm. This method of carrying frees one of your hands for another activity.

"In arms" or *cradle position* (Figure 5-2): The infant's back and head are supported by your left arm (if you are right-handed). For small infants, your left hand can grasp the infant's left thigh; thus freeing your right hand.

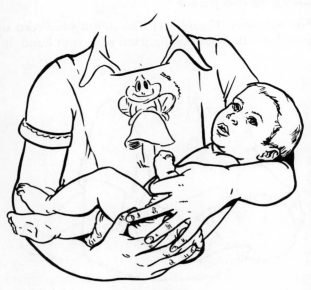

Figure 5-2.

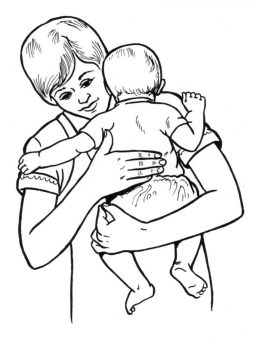

Figure 5-3.

Shoulder carry (Figure 5-3): This position always requires two hands. Place the infant upright, supporting his back with your hand.

Positioning for Procedures

Positioning the child properly for procedures is necessary both for the child's safety during the procedure and to assure the success of the procedure. Always explain (to the parents, if the child himself is too young to understand) what is happening and why the procedure is necessary.

Lumbar puncture (Figure 5-4): Place the child on his side, facing you. Hold him close to the far edge of the table; flex his neck and knees and hold them securely in this position (as shown). To assure that the older infant or child does not move, it may be necessary to wrap his legs in a bath blanket before

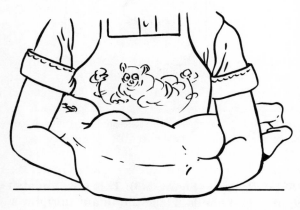

Figure 5-4.

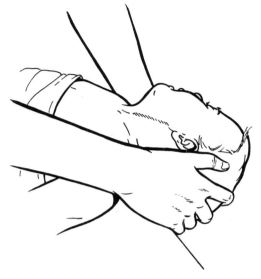

Figure 5-5.

attempting to position him. Observe for signs of respiratory distress while the child is in this position, since his trachea may occlude when his neck is flexed. It is not usually necessary for the child to be kept flat after a spinal tap unless his condition (or doctor's orders) contraindicates activity.

Jugular puncture (Figure 5-5): With the child in a mummy restraint, position his head in hyperextension over the edge of the table. Stabilize his head as shown, being careful not to put pressure over his ears.

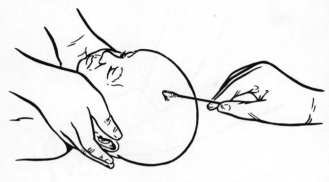

Figure 5-6.

Scalp vein, subdural, or ventricular taps (Figure 5-6): With the child in mummy restraint, hold his head steady between your hands, being careful not to apply pressure over his ears.

Femoral puncture (Figure 5-7): Place the child on his back, with his legs in frogleg position. Restrain his arms with gentle pressure from your arms and hold his legs securely at the knees. Note diaper (indicated by dotted lines) to protect puncture site ("X"), nurse, and physician from urine.

Perineal or rectal procedures (Figure 5-8): With the child on his back, hold his legs in thigh flexion-abduction position. (Dotted line indicates diaper.)

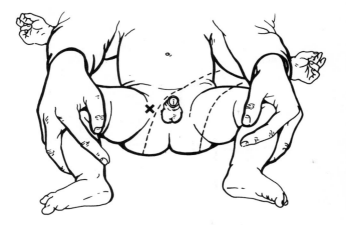

Figure 5-7.

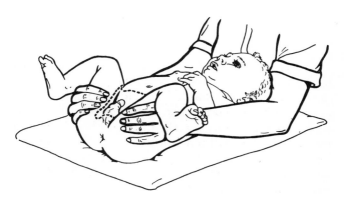

Figure 5-8.

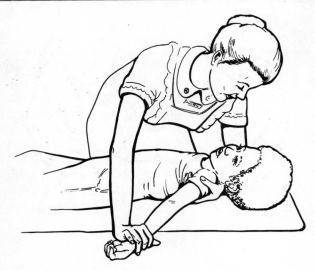

Figure 5-9.

Venipuncture (Figure 5-9): With the child on his back, reach behind his neck and hold his left shoulder with your left hand. The child's right arm is secured behind your back. Reach across the child and hold his left wrist with your right hand. He will be able to kick without interfering with the procedure, and he can hug you with his right arm when he is in pain. Your face will be in alignment with his; this allows verbal and nonverbal interaction during the procedure.

RESTRAINTS

Restraints are a necessary part of the nursing of children, but they are used as a last resort and must never take the place of careful nursing observations. They are used to protect the child from injury and to facilitate examinations and treatments. Restraints must be applied correctly to avoid circulatory impairment, skin irritation, and unnecessary restrictions of movement. Adequately pad restraints to protect the skin and place the child in correct body alignment. Tie all restraints to the bed frame, never to the side rails. All knots used should be such that they can be easily released.

Check restraints every 15 minutes (including circulatory checks of the restrained limb), and remove them every one to two hours to permit movement. Observe the child carefully when his restraints are removed so that he does not injure himself (e.g., by pulling out his IV or nasogastric tubing).

Mummy Restraint

The mummy restraint is used for procedures involving the neck or head; for example, jugular punctures, beginning scalp-vein infusions, and insertion of nasogastric tubes.

Procedure

As shown in Figure 5-10 place blanket on bed; fold down one corner (A). Place the child on his back on the blanket with his shoulder at the fold.

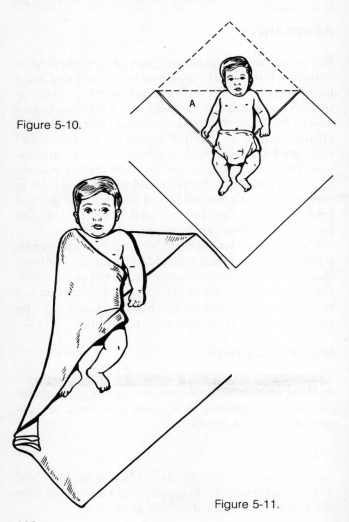

Figure 5-10.

A

Figure 5-11.

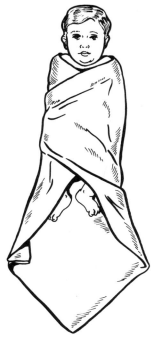

Figure 5-12.

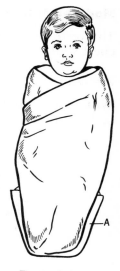

Figure 5-13.

With the child's right arm in a comfortable position, fold blanket over the arm and across the abdomen; tuck snugly behind back (Figure 5-11).

Repeat for left arm as shown in Figure 5-12.

Figure 5-13 illustrates the excess blanket tucked under the child (A). It also can be brought up over his abdomen and the sides tucked under his back (see Figure 5-16).

Modified Mummy Restraint

This restraint is used for procedures on the anterior chest wall.

Procedure

With blanket folded in a rectangle, place the child on longitudinal fold, shoulders level with fold (Fig-

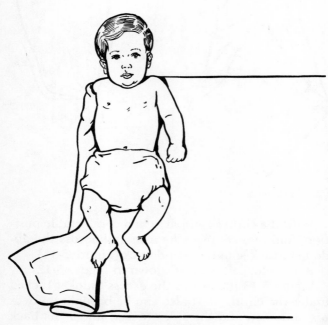

Figure 5-14.

ure 5-14). His arm is positioned comfortably at his side. Fold the blanket over the arm, and tuck it snugly under child's back.

Repeat for the other arm (Figure 5-15).

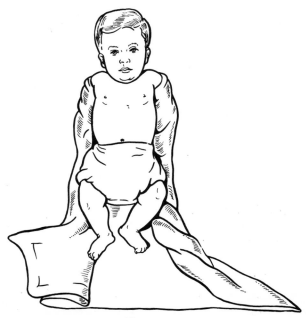

Figure 5-15.

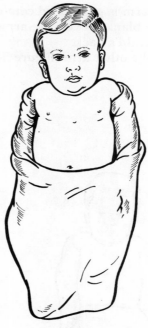

Figure 5-16.

Bring the excess up over the abdomen and, leaving chest exposed, secure sides of blanket behind child's back (Figure 5-16).

Elbow Restraint

This method of restraint is used to prevent flexion of the elbow; for example, to prevent the child with a cleft-lip repair from damaging his suture line or to prevent dislodgement of a scalp-vein infusion. This restraint consists of a piece of material with pockets sewn to accommodate tongue blades. The number of tongue blades inserted depends on the size of the child's arm.

Procedure

Figure 5-17 illustrates the elbow restraint. Insert tongue blades in restraint (*a*). If full-length tongue blades are too long for the child, cut them to correct size with your scissors. Fold the restraint down over the tongue blades to assure a proper fit. Pad the child's arm with shirt sleeve or other soft material (*b*), and wrap the restraint around his arm. Tie or pin the restraint securely (*c*). Be sure that the restraint does not rub child's axilla or wrist.

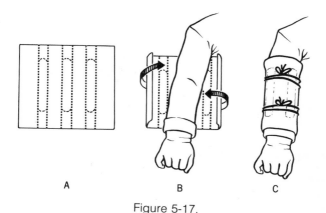

A   B   C

Figure 5-17.

Clove-Hitch Restraint

The clove hitch is an extremity restraint. It is always padded, usually with the child's shirt sleeve or a gauze square. The clove hitch is *not* a slipknot; if properly applied, it will not tighten and interfere with circulation. Always anchor it to the bed frame, not to the side rails.

Equipment

Three- or four-foot length of two-inch gauze, folded lengthwise.
Padding for wrist or ankle.

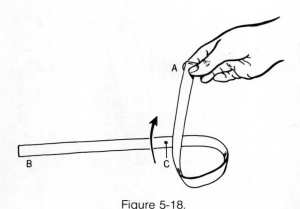

Figure 5-18.

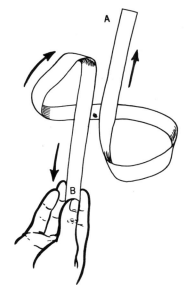

Figure 5-19.

Procedure for Clove-Hitch Restraint

With gauze on flat surface, bring (A) over center point (C). (See Figure 5-18.) Bring (B) over center point in opposite direction to make a figure eight. (Figure 5-19.)

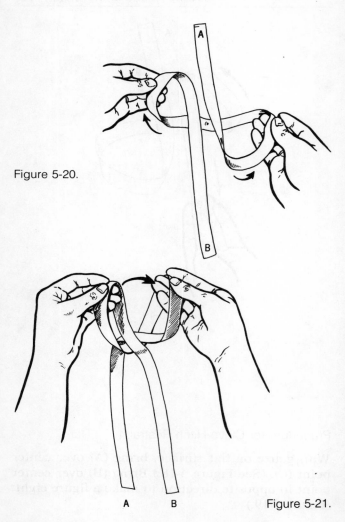

Figure 5-20.

Figure 5-21.

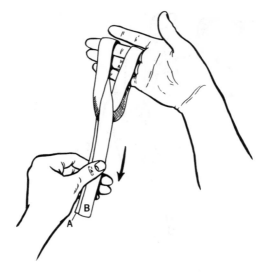

Figure 5-22.

Pick up both loops, bringing hands together (Figure 5-20). Place both loops on one hand (Figure 5-21). With other hand, pull (A) and (B) firmly (Figure 5-22).

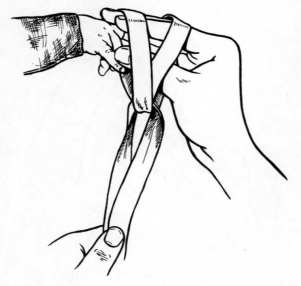

Figure 5-23.

Slip clove hitch over child's hand or foot, onto wrist or ankle. (See Figure 5-23.)

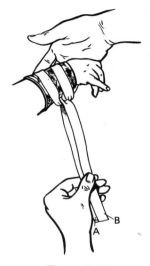

Figure 5-24.

Tighten knot around wrist or ankle by pulling ends (A) and (B) alternately and firmly (Figure 5-24). The knot should be tight enough so that it does not slip off the hand and loose enough so that circulation is not impaired. You can place the tip of your little finger between the child's arm and the gauze if the knot is tied correctly.

Jacket Restraint

To keep the child in bed, high chair, or wheelchair a jacket restraint is used.

This halter-type restraint (Figure 5-25) is tied at the back to keep the child from removing it. The long ties are secured to bed frame. The child may move around in bed, but he cannot climb out. Check him often to see that he does not become entangled in the long ties.

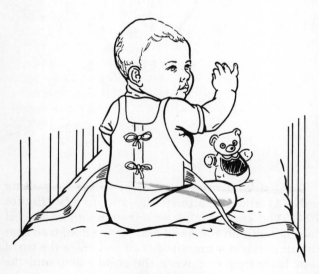

Figure 5-25.

CAST CARE

The child in a cast requires meticulous nursing care. Many complications are directly caused by poor nursing care and can be prevented. Precast neurovascular status in all four extremities should be evaluated, if possible, to serve as a baseline for future comparisons.

During cast application, a stockinette is stretched over the area to be casted; bony prominences are padded with cotton sheeting. Rolls of gauze impregnated with plaster of paris are soaked in cold water and then applied to the extremity. As the cast dries, heat is produced by a chemical reaction between the plaster and the water. Explain this both to the child and to the parents so that they will not think the cast is burning him. Support the wet cast with plastic-covered pillows and handle it with the palms of your hands. (Fingers may cause indentations in the cast, producing pressure areas.) When the cast is dry, it will have a hollow sound when tapped with the fingers. "Hot spots" on the cast surface usually indicate infection beneath the cast and should be reported immediately. The physician will cut a "window" in the cast so that the area can be observed. After the cast has been applied, elevate the extremity to reduce local edema. (If it is not elevated, the cast can act as a tourniquet.) If edema is excessive, the cast will be bivalved (cut in half longitudinally); the anterior and posterior portions will be held together with an elastic bandage. If an open reduction has been performed, expect bleeding after surgery. Outline the blood-stained area on the cast with a ballpoint pen and mark the time and date. This will serve as a guide for assessing the amount of bleeding.

Neurovascular Assessment

Neurovascular assessments are necessary after cast application. Check every hour for 24 hours or until neurovascular status has returned to normal. Assess all extremities affected by the cast. If the cast

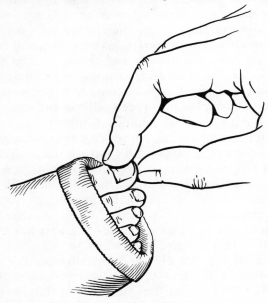

Figure 5-26.

involves the trunk, assess all extremities. Monitor peripheral pulses and assess for increase in pain, cold, edema, and cyanosis.

Press on nail bed to check capillary filling, an indication of circulatory status (Figure 5-26). After the pressure is released, color should rapidly return to normal. Feel the fingers or toes for warmth or coolness. If edema is present, the color is usually poor, the skin cool, and the capillary filling sluggish. If one of these symptoms is detected, elevate the extremity more to prevent progression of other symptoms.

Check sensation and movement by asking the child (if he is over 10) if he can feel pressure or if he can wiggle his fingers or toes. Sensation and movement in the child under 10 should be tested by pinprick. If he feels the prick, he will either cry or move his fingers or toes. Accurately record and report your findings. Avoid ambiguous terms such as "good," "fair," or "poor." Record actual findings, such as "fingers pink, warm to touch; no edema, capillary filling rapid; responds to pinprick with crying and movement of fingers."

Skin Care

The objective of skin care around the cast edges is to toughen the skin and, therefore, to reduce irritation. Apply 70 percent isopropyl alcohol to the skin around the cast edges every four hours. If redness is noticed, increase alcohol application to every hour until redness disappears. Alleviate pressure on the reddened area. Because alcohol is drying, flaking of the skin may be noted. If so, discontinue alcohol application until flaking has stopped. *Do not* use lotions or oils to lubricate the skin because they serve to soften skin and increase the possibility of breakdown. Powders tend to cake and will also cause skin irritation. Skin care to bony prominences and joints is also given every four hours.

Itching under the cast is a common problem. A gauze scratcher may be placed next to the skin, under the stockinette, to aid in relieving itching (Figure 5-27). When it becomes soiled, tie a new piece of gauze to the old piece and pull it through the cast. Caution the child and his parents not to put anything into the cast to scratch because this may cause skin breakdown. Use a fan or aseptic

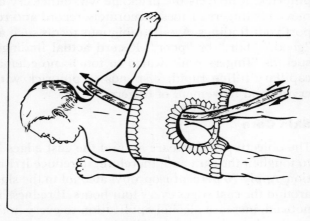

Figure 5-27.

syringe to blow air into the cast to relieve itching, if necessary.

When feeding the child, place a towel over cast edges to prevent crumbs from dropping into cast. Inspect the cast frequently to assure that the child has not placed small items under it. Caution parents to observe the child closely to prevent him from placing small objects under cast.

As cast dries, feel it for tightness. You should be able to place your fingers between cast and skin after it has dried, otherwise cast is too tight and physician should be notified. All casts should be petaled either with stockinette or tape to prevent skin irritation from rough edges. Petaling also prevents the young child from pulling the padding out of the cast.

Figure 5-28 shows cast edges protected with stockinette. During application of cast, stockinette is pulled out over edges of cast and secured 1.25 to 2.5 centimeters (½ to 1 inch) below edge (on outside of cast) with additional plaster of paris (or other casting material).

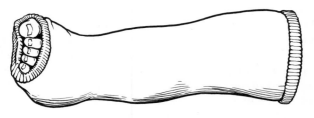

Figure 5-28.

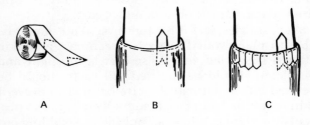

Figure 5-29.

If stockinette padding has not been applied, petaling with adhesive tape is done routinely as soon as the cast is dry (Figure 5-29). Cut 5 to 7.5 centimeter (2 to 3 inch) strips of 2.5-centimeter (1-inch) wide adhesive tape. Ends may be pointed or rounded (square ends tend to curl). Cut a large number of strips before beginning. Insert tape inside cast and bring out over cast edge, pressing firmly to secure tape to cast. Continue applying adhesive strips to cast edge, overlapping each piece to form a smooth edge.

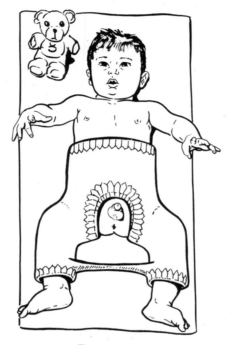

Figure 5-30.

Figure 5-30 depicts a hip spica cast. Note that all edges have been petaled with adhesive. Abduction stabilizer bar between legs is never used as a handle to turn the child.

Positioning and Turning

Casting produces pressure on the skin, especially over bony prominences and joints. Change the child's position at least every four hours; if he has a history of pressure problems or a condition that tends to promote skin problems (meningomyelocele, e.g.), change his position every hour. Support the cast and dependent parts with pillows to assure comfort and prevent pressure sores.

Procedure

Short arm cast (Figure 5-31). The child is positioned on his side with pillows supporting his back, cast,

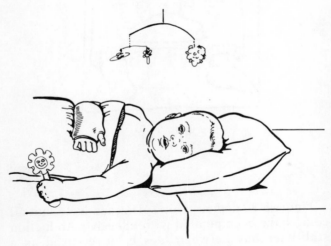

Figure 5-31.

and head. He may be turned from side to supine to prone position.

Positioning child with short arm cast in wheelchair (Figure 5-32). The child's arm is supported with pillows and is elevated higher than the shoulder to prevent edema.

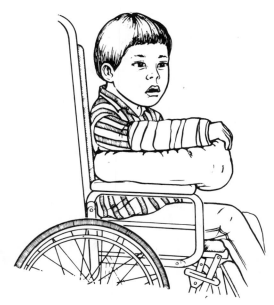

Figure 5-32.

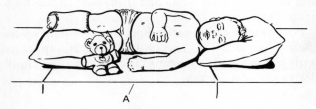

Figure 5-33.

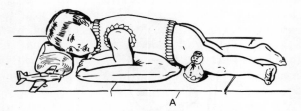

Figure 5-34.

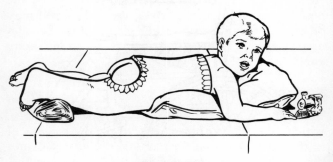

Figure 5-35.

Short leg cast (Figure 5-33). The child is positioned on side with pillows supporting his back, leg, and head. Note draw sheet (A) and snap pants, which are more easily removed than elastic pants which have to be pulled up over the cast. The child may be turned to his back, but the position may be uncomfortable for him.

Risser localizer cast (Figure 5-34). The child is in prone position, with cast supported by pillow; his head is supported by blanket roll (or firm pillow). Because of pressure on the throat, the child usually tolerates this position for only an hour b.i.d. Note draw sheet. The child may be turned to back and both sides, with adequate support for cast and other body parts. With the child in a body cast, observe chest expansion, respiratory rate, color, and behavior.

Hip spica cast (Figure 5-35). Place the child in a prone position, with a pillow placed lengthwise from head to waist. Note the blanket roll used to elevate the right foot (incorporated into cast) off the bed, thus avoiding pressure on toes. The child may be turned to back and either side as long as adequate support is provided to cast and other body parts.

Protecting the Cast

Wetting and soiling of the cast causes it to soften, which may compromise the desired position of immobility. Wet padding under the cast will not dry completely because of the limited circulation.

This continual dampness predisposes the child to skin irritation, infection, or urine dermatitis, which may result in early cast removal and unnecessary hospitalization. Casts are usually soiled either during eating or elimination. At mealtimes, cover the cast with a towel and stay with the child to be sure he does not spill (or deliberately place) food into the cast.

Perineal protection is more difficult to achieve, especially if the child is not toilet trained. For the older child, cover the cast edges nearest the perineum with plastic covering during toileting, and elevate the head of the bed, placing the shoulders higher than the buttocks. This position prevents urine from running back under the cast. After toileting, remove plastic covering.

The child who is not toilet trained needs to have the cast (around the perineum) covered continuously. The covering is removed only when it is soiled and is immediately replaced with clean plastic. Oil of silk, plastic wrap, or plastic garbage bags may be used to protect the cast. Tuck plastic under petaled cast edges and bring it to the outside; secure with adhesive tape and change as necessary.

Procedure

Disposable diaper can be used to keep feces and urine from soiling the cast (Figure 5-36). Separate absorbent diaper pad from plastic backing, *a*; remove adhesive tabs; fold plastic backing in half lengthwise. Fold bottom third of diaper back and place in center of plastic; fold top and bottom of

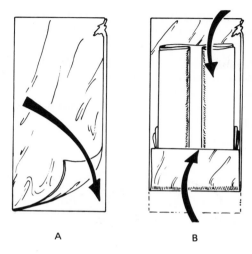

A   B

Figure 5-36.

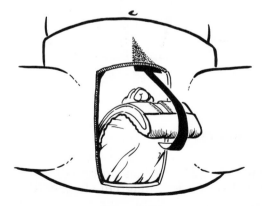

Figure 5-37.

plastic up over pad, *b*. Tuck bottom of the diaper into back of cast (Figure 5-37); bulky portion is tucked under top of cast.

Keep diaper in place with heavy-duty ¾-inch elastic strap with Velcro fasteners (Figure 5-38).

A sanitary pad may also be used to absorb urine and feces, provided the perineal area of the cast is protected with plastic.

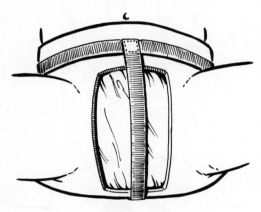

Figure 5-38.

Cast Removal

Removal of the cast is terrifying to the child because the cast cutter makes a frightening noise, and the child believes he will be cut along with the cast. The cast cutter works by vibration and cuts only the hard surface of the cast.

TRACTION CARE

Traction is used in the treatment of fractures to reduce the fracture and to stabilize the site. For traction to be effective, countertraction and friction are necessary. Traction is applied by weights that pull on the distal bone fragment. Body weight serves as countertraction. Friction is the force between the child and the bed.

Muscle spasms or contractions contribute to malalignment of the bone ends. For this reason, traction must be constantly maintained until the muscles are completely relaxed. The stress of traction causes a buildup of lactic acid, which promotes muscle relaxation; then the bone ends can be properly aligned. This realignment process usually takes less time in the infant than it does in the older child because his muscle tone is not as fully developed.

Skin traction is applied directly to the skin and is used when bone displacement is minimal and there is little muscle spasticity. It is not used when there is soft tissue damage. Traction straps are secured to the extremity with elastic bandages or traction tapes; then attached to a foot plate, or spreader. The extremity weight is connected to the footplate to provide pull. When *adhesive* traction straps are used, the nurse never releases the traction; however, when *nonadhesive* straps are used, the nurse may remove the traction as specified by the physician (usually at designated intervals).

Skeletal traction exerts pull by means of a pin or wire inserted through bone. It is used when a stronger pull than can be obtained by skin traction is needed, or when skin traction is contraindicated due to soft tissue damage. Skeletal traction is never released by the nurse.

Skin care must be given at least every four hours. Seventy percent isopropyl alcohol is used to toughen the skin. Restraints are removed for 15 minutes every four hours while alcohol is applied and general skin care is given.

Pin or wire care is given per physician's order. Observe pins and wires for slippage or breakage. If either end of the pin or wire is exposed, cover it with a cork to prevent injury to the child and/or others.

Neurovascular Assessment

Neurovascular assessments are imperative for the child in traction. With meticulous nursing care, impairment can be detected before permanent damage results. Assess neurovascular status before traction is applied to serve as a baseline for future assessments. If there is edema at the site, a "normal" baseline assessment may be impossible to obtain. If so, obtain a verbal assessment from the parents.

Skeletal traction and *skin traction with adhesive* require hourly checks for the first 24 hours, then every four hours (for the duration of traction therapy), if the status has returned to normal. For *nonadhesive* skin traction, neurovascular checks are done every four hours and 30 minutes after the limb has been rewrapped and the traction reapplied. If the limb is wrapped too loosely or too tightly, rewrap, and assess again in 30 minutes.

Procedure

To assess neurovascular status (Figure 5-39), press on nailbed (A); nail should blanch. Release; color should return rapidly if circulation is not sluggish. Test the child's sensation and movement at the same time by using a pinprick (B). The small child may cry and move his toes or fingers away from the prick; the older child may report that he feels the prick. Do not rely on the report of the child under age 10 that he feels the sensation; always test with a pinprick.

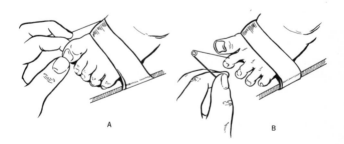

Figure 5-39.

Upper Extremity Traction

Dunlop traction, for fractures and contractures of the elbow, and for postoperative immobilization (Figure 5-40). The elbow is flexed and pull is in two directions: one in direct line with upper arm and one in line with lower arm. Both pelvic and thoracic sling restraints are used to prevent child from sliding toward the affected side.

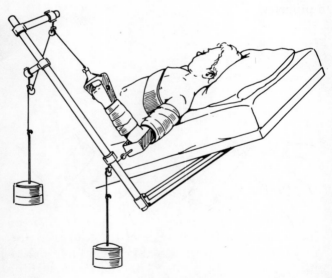

Figure 5-40.

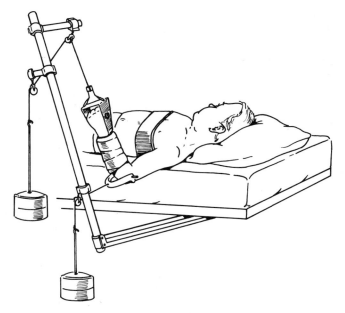

Figure 5-41.

Dunlop with skeletal traction (Figure 5-41). A pin placed through the condyles of the humerus provides traction to upper arm. Skin traction provides pull to lower arm. Both pelvic and thoracic sling restraints are used.

Lower Extremity Traction

Bryant's traction (Figure 5-42). Adhesive skin traction is used for a fractured femur in the child less than two years of age (weighing 12 to 14 kilograms or 26 to 30 pounds). Bryant's traction is not used for the older child because of the danger of postural hypertension and impairment of circulation caused by the increased weight.

Child is supine, with both legs suspended perpendicular to his body. The child's weight provides countertraction; buttocks are slightly elevated

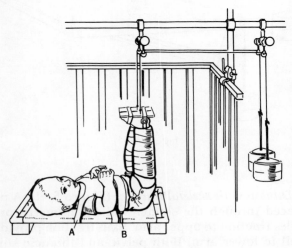

Figure 5-42.

above bed. Both legs are suspended to aid in immobilization even though only one is fractured, and the child is placed on a solid Bradford frame. Note pelvic sling restraint (**A**) and frame restraint (**B**).

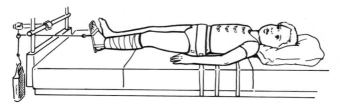

Figure 5-43.

Buck's extension (Figure 5-43). Skin traction with lower extremity in extended position is used to correct hip and knee contractures; to rest the leg in Legg-Calvé-Perthes' disease, for instance, and for other short-term immobilizations. The child may be placed prone or supine and may be turned to the side, provided the affected leg is kept in alignment. Note pelvic sling and jacket restraints, and draw sheet.

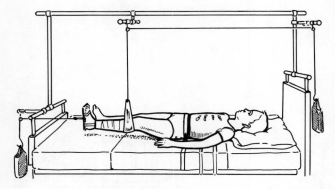

Figure 5-44.

Split Russell traction (Figure 5-44) is used to reduce contractures of the hip or knee, to immobilize and rest the hip or knee postoperatively, and to reduce dislocated hips. A supine position is used, with skin traction to lower leg exerting longitudinal pull, and a sling under the proximal tibia or knee exerting perpendicular or vertical pull. A wire or pin may be used in the distal femur if necessary. Jacket restraint is used if skeletal pin or wire is used; otherwise, a pelvic sling restraint (not shown) is necessary.

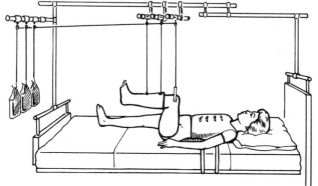

Figure 5-45.

Ninety-degree—90-degree traction (90—90 trac-tion) (Figure 5-45) is used for fractured femur when skin traction is not adequate to reduce the fracture. Both knee and hip are flexed at a 90 degree angle. A short leg "boot" cast is used to suspend the lower leg, and a pin or wire is inserted through the distal femur to apply skeletal traction to the thigh. A pelvic sling restraint and jacket restraint are both necessary, and if immobilization problems are anticipated, the opposite leg may be placed in split Russell traction.

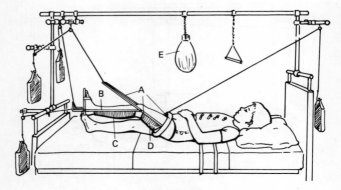

Figure 5-46.

Balance suspension with Thomas ring splint (**A**) and *Pearson attachment* (**B**) (Figure 5-46) is used for older children and adolescents for fractured femurs, resting the hip and knee, and postoperative hip and knee immobilization. Canvas or stockinette (**C**) covers the Pearson attachment and Thomas splint (**D**) to support the leg. Note jacket restraint and draw sheet; the punching bag (**E**) is to help child release aggression.

Cervical Traction

Procedure

Cervical traction, applied by means of head halter attached to pulley at end of bed, is used for muscle spasms and cervical injuries (Figure 5-47). The head is in neutral position and head of bed is elevated 15 to 20 degrees. A pelvic sling is necessary.

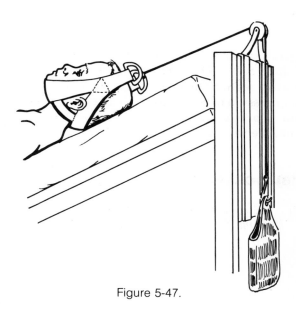

Figure 5-47.

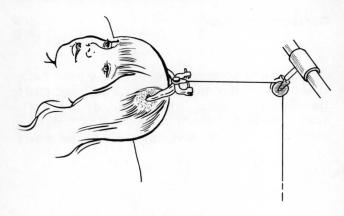

Figure 5-48.

Crutchfield tongs applied to skull via burr holes (Figure 5-48). This method of skeletal traction is used to reduce fractures of cervical vertebrae and compression of spinal cord. Head is hyperextended, and a pelvic sling restraint is used to help immobilize the child.

BIBLIOGRAPHY

Hill, N.E. and Schmitt, E.W. Jr. *Pediatric Orthopedic Nursing.* St. Louis, C.V. Mosby Co., 1975.

CHAPTER 6

Fluid and Electrolyte Needs of the Child

SPECIMEN COLLECTION

Urine Collection

Because catheterization can introduce bacteria into the bladder, a clean-catch, midstream specimen is usually preferred for urine cultures. The perineal area must be washed well with soap and water to minimize contamination of voided urine by organisms on the skin.

Equipment

Sterile cotton balls
Sterile water
Antiseptic solution
Soap
Sterile specimen container
Urine collection bag

Procedure for Urine Collection

For girls, separate the labia, and use a soapy cotton ball to wash from clitoris to anus on one side of urinary meatus (see Figure 2-6, page 51). Repeat on other side with a second cotton ball; with a third cotton ball, wash directly over the meatus. Rinse in the same manner, using three more cotton balls saturated with sterile water. Repeat entire procedure using an antiseptic solution, sterile water to rinse, and dry cotton balls to dry. Have the child begin to void into the toilet; then place a sterile urine cup into stream to catch midstream specimen.

For boys, wash the penis, using a circular motion toward the scrotum, remembering to retract foreskin if the child is not circumcised (see Figure 2-8, page 52). Collect specimen the same way as for girls. The older boy can cleanse his own penis if properly instructed.

Obtaining a urine specimen from an infant requires the use of a urine collection bag such as the U-Bag collector by Hollister, shown in the following figures. Before applying the bag, be sure the infant's genitals are clean and dry, following the instructions given above.

Remove protective paper from bottom half of adhesive patch (Figure 6-1). Stretch the infant's legs apart to separate skin folds. Fit the collector over vagina or penis and scrotum (Figure 6-2), then press adhesive to skin, starting at narrow bridge of skin separating the anus from the genitals. Work outward, firmly pressing adhesive as you go. When

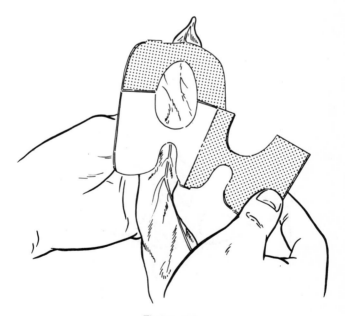

Figure 6-1.

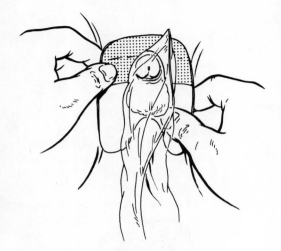

Figure 6-2.

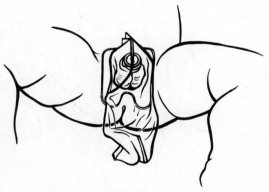

Figure 6-3.

bottom part of adhesive is in place, remove backing from top part of adhesive patch, and press firmly against skin, avoiding wrinkles.

Urine collection bag in place (Figure 6-3). The child may be diapered to keep urine bag in place.

If a 24-hour urine bag is used, it will have a length of tubing attached to it which can be connected to a bedside receptacle (Figure 6-4). However, to allow the child freedom of movement, you can shorten tube, (*a*); attach plastic junction, (*b*); and apply cap, (*c*). Curl the tubing into the diaper, and the child can be up and out of bed. To reconnect both ends of tubing, remove cap *c* and attach remaining length of tube to plastic junction *b*. After the child has voided, or after a 24-hour specimen has been collected, gently remove the bag, wash the perineal area, and rediaper the infant. Note condition of skin where bag was applied.

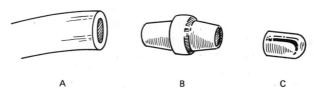

A   B   C

Figure 6-4.

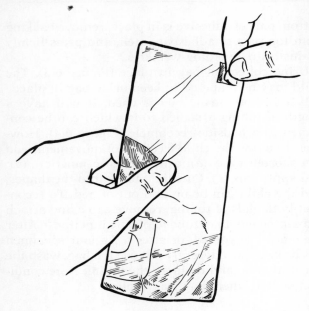

Figure 6-5.

To drain urine into the specimen bottle, invert the bag and remove blue tab from the lower corner, being careful not to spill urine (Figure 6-5).

Pour urine into specimen bottle (Figure 6-6). Label properly, record amount and color of urine, and send specimen to laboratory.

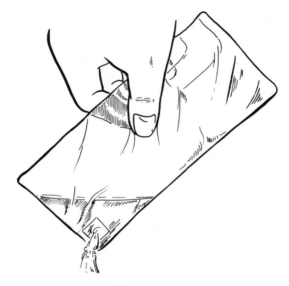

Figure 6-6.

Stool Collection

Equipment

Diaper
Cellophane or plastic
Tongue blade
Specimen container

Procedure for Stool Collection

For soft or formed stool, scrape a small amount of stool from diaper with tongue blade. Place in specimen cup, label, and send to laboratory.

If stools are diarrheal (watery or loose), place a piece of cellophane or plastic between child and diaper to catch stool (Figure 6-7), otherwise it will be absorbed into the diaper. Transfer stool from cellophane directly into specimen cup. Label and send to laboratory; record amount, character, and consistency of stool.

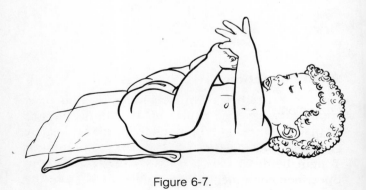

Figure 6-7.

ENEMAS

Enemas are used to cleanse the colon before diagnostic or surgical procedures involving the bowels.
An enema is uncomfortable and potentially
dangerous. Hard plastic enema tips can perforate
the rectum, so a soft rubber catheter is preferred.
Because tap water can be absorbed and cause
water intoxication, it is not used as an enema solution; rather, normal saline, or milk, is preferred. A
stimulating suppository combined with an oral
cathartic is effective for emptying the colon and is
tolerated better by the child than is an enema.

Equipment

Enema solution
    Soapsuds: 8 ml soap jelly to 500 ml water
    Saline: 4 ml salt to 500 ml water
Catheter (size 12 to 16 French for infants; 24 to 30
for older children)
Reservoir
Plastic sheeting
Bedpan

Procedure

Place infant supine on pillows to support his back
and head, with his buttocks on a small bedpan (or
on plastic sheeting) (Figure 6-8). Secure his legs by
placing a diaper under the bedpan and pinning it
around his thighs. (An alternative method is to pin
the diaper ends around his thighs, then bring the

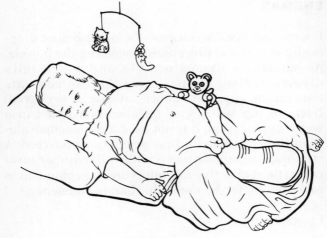

Figure 6-8.

middle up and pin it to his diaper shirt). The older child may be placed on his left side with his right leg flexed.

Insert a catheter 3.7 to 10 centimeters (1½ to 4 inches) into rectum (just within the anal sphincter). Hang reservoir with warmed solution 30 to 45 centimeters (12 to 18 inches) above the infant's hips, and allow solution to run in by gravity. The amount of solution will vary from 30 to 300 milliliters (1 to 10 ounces) depending on the size of the child.

Never administer more than 300 milliliters to an infant unless ordered by physician. Allow the child to expel solution into bedpan, potty chair, or plastic sheeting, depending on his age and condition. If solution is to be retained, hold or tape buttocks together and keep child as quiet as possible.

Colonic irrigation is used to empty the bowel; for example, in Hirschsprung's disease. The child may be placed on his left side with knees flexed, or positioned on a bedpan as illustrated (Figure 6-9). The irrigation solution is placed in large syringe attached to a soft catheter. Lubricate the catheter tip and insert it with a twirling motion, injecting as you insert. This prevents bowel perforation because the stream of liquid diverts the catheter tip away from bowel wall. Inject fluid, then aspirate solution and feces, repeating until the return is clear of fecal material.

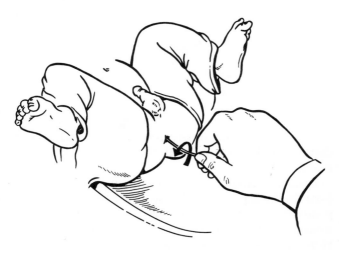

Figure 6-9.

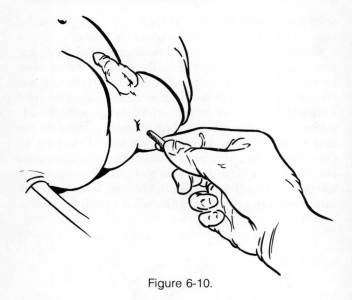

Figure 6-10.

Discontinue and notify physician if abdominal distention increases or if the child experiences pain.

Inserting a suppository is illustrated in Figure 6-10. Using a gloved hand or finger cot, insert suppository into rectum, pushing it beyond the internal anal sphincter to prevent immediate expulsion. Hold or tape the child's buttocks together and keep him quiet.

OSTOMY CARE

Colostomy and ileostomy care in the infant are often complicated by the small size of the stoma; standard appliances are not made small enough for the tiny infant. The infant's skin is fragile, and breakdown from drainage can occur rapidly. In addition, the stools of the infant with a stoma are more liquid than the adult's, primarily because of the infant's diet. When a newborn requires a stoma, his routine care is complicated by the fact that the parents not only must learn to care for their new baby but also must learn special-care techniques because his bowel empties on the surface of his abdomen. The parents need a great deal of support and understanding, even if the stoma is temporary, which is usually the case.

Postoperatively, wound contamination is a possibility until the incision has healed. A dry sterile dressing is placed over the incision, and the stoma is left uncovered until peristalsis returns and the child begins passing stools (about 24 hours). Never place one large dressing over incision and stoma. Restrain the child so that he does not kick or bump the fresh stoma, which bleeds easily.

Irrigations, to help regulate bowel movements, are not routinely done on the child with a colostomy. However, the physician may dilate the stoma to check for bowel stenosis, to widen the stomal lumen, and to encourage passage of stool. Saline soaks, alternated with petroleum-jelly impregnated gauze, which is changed when soiled, are used to keep the stoma soft and to prevent crusting caused by excessive drainage. Skin care to prevent excoriation around the stoma consists of keeping the skin clean and dry. Inspection of the site for signs of irritation or inflammation is essential, even before peristalsis returns and dressings are applied.

Equipment

Zinc oxide
Tissue paper
Twill tape or umbilical ligature
Adhesive tape
Tincture of benzoin
Karaya gum powder
Collecting device

Procedure

Zinc oxide and tissue-paper dressing are used for protecting skin around stoma from drainage for infants too small for commercial collecting devices (Figure 6-11). The dressing is absorbent, nonirritating, and can be adapted as the infant grows by varying the size of the tissue square and adding extra layers of tissue for absorbency.

Fold tissue in half until it forms a two-inch square. Cut a hole slightly larger than the stoma in the center of the tissue. Apply a thick layer of zinc oxide around stoma, working outward to protect surrounding skin area from the corrosive action of

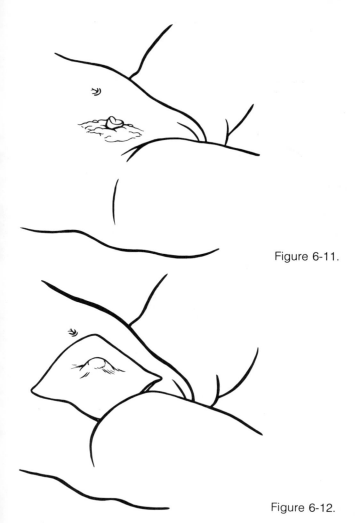

Figure 6-11.

Figure 6-12.

digestive enzymes in the liquid stool that is characteristic of ileostomy patients.

Apply fitted tissue over zinc oxide to absorb drainage (Figure 6-12). Cover with another folded two-inch square of tissue, which acts as an absorbent pad for stool collection.

Secure dressing with Montgomery straps (Figure 6-13). Change dressing at least every two to three hours, clean area, inspect for irritation, and reapply dressing. Record frequency, color, and consistency of stools as well as condition of skin.

Excessive diarrhea or liquid stools contribute to skin breakdown. In such cases, apply tincture of benzoin around stoma and sprinkle with karaya

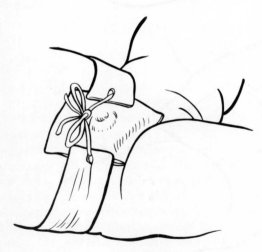

Figure 6-13.

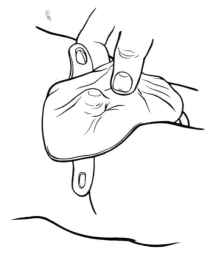

Figure 6-14.

gum powder to aid healing and prevent further breakdown. Proceed with zinc-oxide dressing.

When using an ostomy bag, form a tight seal around the stoma to prevent leakage onto the skin (Figure 6-14). Cleanse skin around stoma meticulously, then paint a two- to three-inch radius with tincture of benzoin. Cut karaya gum washer to fit snugly around stoma. Paint one side of washer with benzoin and apply this side to skin. Apply ostomy bag with its own karaya gum seal over the stoma and washer to create a tight double seal that is contoured to both abdomen and stoma, thus providing greater protection.

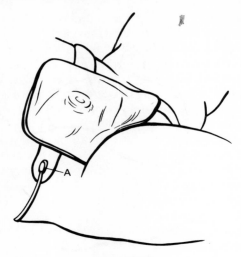

Figure 6-15.

Secure bag with diaper or twill-tape ties attached to belt hooks (A) on ostomy bag (Figure 6-15). Change the bag every 24 hours when you bathe and weigh the infant.

INTRAVENOUS INFUSIONS

Intravenous fluid therapy often is used for the child who is unable to take nourishment orally or who has a fluid and electrolyte imbalance. IVs are also used to administer medications. The fluid-therapy intake is calculated in 24-hour blocks to maintain the child's urine output in the normal range for his age. Bottles containing no more than 250 milliliters are used for the child under five years of age. No more than 500 milliliters per bottle are used on any child to avoid accidental overload.

Special pediatric administration sets, with calibrated volume chambers that hold only 100 to 150 milliliters of fluid at one time, are used to minimize the possibility of errors. These sets deliver 50 or 60 drops/ml as opposed to adult IV sets, which deliver 10, 12, or 15 drops/ml.

Various commonly used intravenous fluids are shown in Table 6-1.

Equipment

Correct fluid per physician's order
Extension tubing
Volume control chamber with microdrip
Filter
Armboard or tongue blade padded with gauze
Tourniquet
Alcohol and Betadine (providone iodine) swabs
One-half-, one-, and two-inch adhesive tape
Needles (usually 21-, 23-, or 25-gauge butterfly needle)
Two-inch gauze squares
Paper or plastic cup with bottom cut out and edges padded with tape
For scalp vein: two rubber bands, safety razor

Table 6-1. Composition of Frequently Used Parenteral Fluids

| Liquid | CHO | Protein* | Cal/L | Na | K | CL | HCO$_3$** | Ca | P† |
	gm/100 ml					mEq/L††			
D$_5$W	5	—	170	—	—	—	—	—	—
D$_{10}$W	10	—	340	—	—	—	—	—	—
Normal Saline (0.9% NaCl)	—	—	—	154	—	154	—	—	—
1/2 Normal Saline (0.45% NaCl)	—	—	—	77	—	77	—	—	—
D$_5$ (0.2% NaCl)	5	—	170	34	—	34	—	—	—
3% Saline	—	—	—	513	—	513	—	—	—
8.4% Sodium Bicarbonate (1 mEq/ml)	—	—	—	1000	—	—	1000	—	—
Ringer's	0–10	—	0–340	147	4	155.5	—	4.5	—
Ringer's Lactate	0–10	—	0–340	130	4	109	28	3	—
Amino Acid 8.5% (Travasol)	—	8.5	340	3	—	34	52	—	—
Plasmanate	—	5	200	110	2	50	29	—	—

Albumin 25% (Salt Poor)	—	25	1000	100–160	<1	<120			—	—	—
Intralipid (Cutter)§	2.25	—	1100		2.6		0.5	4.0	—	—	27

* Protein or amino acid equivalent.
** Bicarbonate or equivalent (citrate, acetate, lactate).
† Calculated according to valence of 1.8.
†† Approximate values: actual values may vary somewhat in various localities depending on electrolyte composition of water supply used to reconstitute solution.
§ Values are approximate—may vary from lot to lot.

Reproduced with permission from Johns Hopkins Hospital. *The Harriet Lane Handbook*, Ed. 8. Kenneth C. Schuberth and Basil J. Zitelli (Eds). Copyright © 1978 by Year Book Medical Publishers, Inc., Chicago.

Calculating Flow Rate

Use the following formula to calculate the flow rate:

$$\frac{\text{Total volume infused}}{\text{Number of hours of infusion}} = \text{ml/hr}$$

For example: The physician orders 250 ml of D_5W to infuse in four hours and the microdrip for your equipment delivers 50 drops/ml:

$$\frac{250 \text{ ml}}{4 \text{ hours}} = 62 \text{ ml/hr}$$

To convert this to drops per minute, use the formula:

$$\frac{\text{ml/hr} \times \text{drops/ml}}{\text{min/hr}} = \text{drops/min}$$

$$\frac{62 \text{ (ml/hr)} \times 50 \text{ (drops/ml)}}{60 \text{ (min/hr)}} = 52 \text{ drops/min}$$

This two-step formula can be combined into one step:

$$\frac{\text{Total volume} \times \text{drops/ml}}{\text{Total infusion time in min}} = \text{drops/min}$$

$$\frac{250 \text{ (ml)} \times 50 \text{ (drops/ml)}}{240 \text{ minutes} \, (4 \text{ hours} \times 60 \text{ minutes})} = 52 \text{ drops/min}$$

The disadvantage of this last formula is that it does not calculate ml/hr, and, because of the difficulty of regulating IV fluids in the child, drops/min may be difficult to control. You must also know the desired volume/hr, which is more easily controlled.

If your equipment delivers 60 drops/ml, the calculation is simple. The drop factor (60/ml) is equal to the number of min/hr (60); therefore, these two figures cancel each other, with the result that "ml/hr" equals "drops/min." Using the same example as above:

$$\frac{250 \text{ ml} \times 60 \text{ drops/ml}}{4 \text{ (hours)} \times 60 \text{ (minutes)}} = 62 \text{ ml/hr or drops/min}$$

If the physician orders the ml/hr, and your equipment is not a microdrip set, figure the drops/minute.

Example: "Run IV at 30 ml/hr." Your equipment delivers 10 drops/ml.

$$\frac{30 \text{ (ml/hr)} \times 10 \text{ (drops/ml)}}{60 \text{ (min/hr)}} = 5 \text{ drops/min}$$

Setting up IV

Figure 6-16 is a pediatric intravenous infusion set: 250 ml bottle (A); open/close control (B); calibrated volume control chamber (C); air vent open/close control (D); medication injection site (E); drip chamber (F); pediatric microdrip (G) (60 drops = 1 ml); flow control clamp (H); Y-injection site for administration of medications (I); filter (J); flashtube for flashback and administration of medication (K); needle adapter (L).

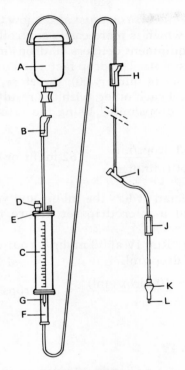

Figure 6-16.

Procedure for Setting Up IV

1. Turn bottle of fluid upside down and hold it up
   to light to inspect for impurities. Solution
   should be clear. Slowly rotate bottle in the

light, observing for bright flashes of reflected light, which indicate cracks in the glass. Do not use solution if it contains obvious impurities or if glass is cracked.

2. Check bottle seal to be sure it has not been broken. If seal has been broken by pharmacist to add medication or electrolytes, bottle should be labeled accordingly. Check labels to see that they match physician's orders.

3. Close clamps on IV tubing.

4. Remove outer cap, metal disc, and rubber disc from fluid bottle.

5. Remove protective cap from spike of infusion set and insert through outlet hole in bottle stopper. Hang IV bottle.

6. Open upper clamp (B) and fill volume control chamber (C) with 30 milliliters of fluid. Close clamp.

7. Gently squeeze drip chamber (F) and fill one third full; this seals tubing at bottom of chamber with liquid and keeps air from entering tubing.

8. Remove protective covering from needle adapter; attach sterile IV needle. Open flow control clamp (H) and run solution through tubing, allowing some fluid to flow from needle. Close clamp.

9. Open upper clamp and fill volume control chamber (C) to desired level (amount ordered per hour plus 10 milliliters for safety or no more than two hours' worth of fluid).

10. Prepare child for procedure, giving him time to ask questions and express his feelings. Restrain him as deemed necessary according to his age, ability to cope with stressful situations, and degree of cooperation. Talk to him throughout procedure, offering support via touch and comforting words. Remember that you are "helping him to hold still," not "holding him down."

11. Assist with or perform venipuncture yourself (according to the policy in your institution), being sure to obtain adequate assistance from another nurse should you start the IV yourself.

12. After venipuncture, secure needle properly to provide easy visibility and maximum mobility while minimizing the risk of dislodging needle. After securing the needle, tape a loop of tubing near insertion site to prevent dislodgment in case tubing is accidentally pulled. Cover site with plastic or paper cup with bottom cut out and edges padded with tape.

13. Adjust flow rate and tape all tubing connections.

14. Attach IV tubing to infusion controller or pump, according to policy in your institution. A wide variety of infusion assistance devices are available; know your equipment and do not confuse monitors or controllers with pumps. Remember that infusion monitors or pumps are never a substitute for your careful observation.

15. Record on pediatric intravenous infusion rec-

Time (Hour)	Bottle Number	Solution	Medication Added	Rate Ordered	Drop Chamber Filled to (ml)	Actual Hourly Intake (ml)	Total Intake (ml)	Desired Intake (ml)	Observed Infusion Site	Comments	Initial
8	1	D5 250 ml.		30 ml/hr	40	32	32	30	✓	Started 7a.m.	Lu
9		E10 MEg KAC			40	32	64	60	OK	left hand	Lu
10			Ampicillin		40	28	92	90	OK		Lu
11			250 mg/5ml		40	30	122	120		puffy md – IV D/c	Lu
12N					40	30	152	150	puffy md – IV D/c	Lu
1											
2											
3											
4											
5											
6											
7											
8											
9											
10											
11											
12MN											
1											
2											
3											
4											
5											
6											
7											

Figure 6-17.

ord, or flow chart (Figure 6-17) the time IV was started, site, type and amount of fluid, rate (ml/hr and drops/min), size of needle used, and amount of fluid in volume chamber. Be sure bottle is properly labeled with child's name, date, and time hung, additives, and your name.

16. Place child on intake and output record, noting daily weights.

IV Sites

Figure 6-18 is a scalp vein infusion. Note that the head is shaved around the site and that a loop of tubing is secured with a second piece of tape. A paper cup is taped over site to protect it. The bottom of the cup has been cut away to permit easy viewing of insertion site (inset).

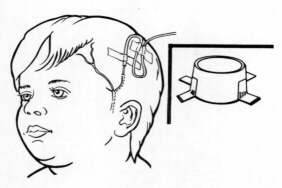

Figure 6-18.

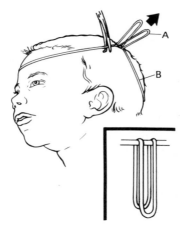

Figure 6-19.

Figure 6-19 shows a rubber band tourniquet for scalp vein infusion. Use two rubber bands; place one crosswise (A and inset) under the band to be used as a tourniquet. Stretch second band (B) around the infant's head to serve as a tourniquet. After venipuncture, grasp (A) and pull, lifting tourniquet (B). Snip the tourniquet with a scissors, holding both ends to keep it from hitting child.

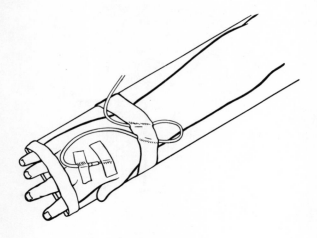

Figure 6-20.

Figure 6-20 depicts an IV in hand. Note the armboard used to keep wrist stable and the loop of tubing secured with second piece of tape.

Figure 6-21 shows an IV in foot (used only in nonwalking children unless absolutely necessary). Note the armboard used to stabilize ankle. The foot is turned medially to expose vein. Be sure the armboard is well padded over bony prominences to prevent pressure sores.

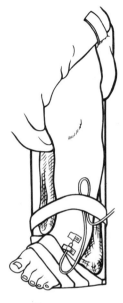

Figure 6-21.

Maintaining IV Infusion

Check rate and site every 30 minutes; record hourly on pediatric intravenous infusion record. During hourly check, be sure to

1. observe site and surrounding tissue for signs of irritation or infiltration.
2. check all tubing connections.
3. check tubing for air bubbles, kinks, and leaks.

4. check amount of fluid in volume control chamber; it should contain no more than two hours' worth of fluid.
5. check that clamp between bottle and control chamber is closed.
6. briefly release all joints for ROM except for joint under IV site.
7. time drip rate for one minute to check accuracy.
8. observe child for signs of discomfort and ask him how IV feels.

BIBLIOGRAPHY

Bishop, W.S. and Head, J.J. Care of the Infant with a Stoma *American Journal of Maternal-Child Nursing* 1:315, 1976.

Mahoney, J.M. What You Should Know About Ostomies *Nursing '78* 8:74, May 1978.

Guhlow, L.J. and Kolb, J. Pediatric IVs: Special Measures You Must Take *RN* 42:40, 1979.

CHAPTER 7

Medicating the Child

SAFE DOSAGE CALCULATION

Although the physician prescribes medications, the nurse has the responsibility for administering most drugs and must know the safe dosage range for all drugs she administers. If, after calculating the safe dosage for the individual child, you feel the prescribed amount is excessive, notify the physician. If he is in error, he will appreciate your intervention; if the dosage is correct, he will explain why he ordered it. If you still doubt the safety of the dosage, consult your nursing supervisor.

Calculations for drug dosage are based on the child's weight or his body surface area (BSA) measured in square meters. Requirements for fluid and electrolytes and therapeutic dosages of many medications are roughly proportional to the BSA, except for neonates and premature infants. Doses based on different criteria may not correspond.

Procedure for Calculating Safe Dosage

Several nomograms and formulas are used to determine BSA. Two methods are offered: a nomogram and a simple formula. After ascertaining the BSA, use this rule to calculate the child's safe dosage:

$$\frac{\text{child's BSA}}{1.7 \text{ (average adult BSA)}} \times \frac{\text{adult}}{\text{dose}} = \frac{\text{child's safe}}{\text{dose}}$$

For example, if the physician orders 100 mg of drug "X," and you know the average adult dose is 250 mg, determine the child's BSA, then use the formula:

$$\frac{0.75 \text{ (child's BSA)}}{1.7 \text{ (adult BSA)}} \times 250 \text{ mg} = \frac{110 \text{ mg}}{\text{(child's safe dose)}}$$

The prescribed dosage of 100 mg is within the child's safe dosage range and may be given.

Figure 7-1 is a nomogram for estimation of body surface area. The surface area is indicated either where a straight line that connects the height (A) and weight (D) levels intersects the surface area column (C) or, if the patient is of average size, from the weight alone (B) (enclosed area). Line (E) represents a child 114 centimeters (45 inches) tall who weighs 20 kilograms (45 pounds); it intersects the surface area column (C) at 0.8 M². The child's BSA is therefore 0.8 square meters. (Nomogram modified from data of E. Boyd by C. D. West. Courtesy of W. B. Saunders Co.)

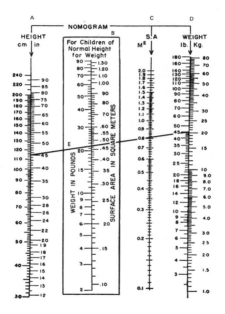

Figure 7-1.

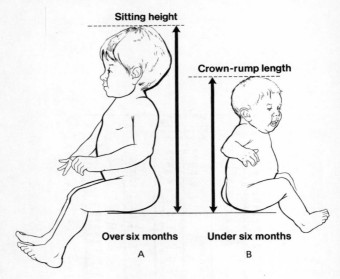

Figure 7-2.

Figure 7-2 shows a quick method for determining BSA in the child under 14½ years of age when nomogram is not available. It requires a centimeter measure.

For the child over six months of age, measure his sitting height in centimeters, as shown a; square this, then multiply by 0.00019 to get child's BSA.

Example: Sitting height is 60 cm:

$$0.00019 \times 60^2 \ (3{,}600) = .68 \ m^2$$

For the infant less than six months of age, measure the crown to rump length as shown *b*, square it, then multiply by 0.00017 to get his BSA.

Example: Crown-rump length is 40 cm:

$$0.00017 \times 40^2 \ (1600) = 0.27\text{m}^2$$

ADMINISTERING MEDICATIONS

Verify the child's identity by checking his armband before giving any medications. Asking a preschooler, "Are you Tammy Smith?" will get a "yes" answer from Peggy, Jimmy, or Gail, all anxious to please, and the older child may deny his identity to escape medication time.

The administration of medications is often viewed as an intrusive procedure by the child. The approach you use in giving medications may convey hostility to the child, and he can, in fact, have the last word by vomiting the medicine.

Use a matter-of-fact approach, such as, "It is time for your medicine." If you give the child a choice about whether or not he is ready for the medicine, he will choose not to be ready. For example, "Are you ready for your injection, Jeff?" or "It's time for your injection, OK?" will elicit a quick "No" response. In this case, you will have to abide by the child's decision and leave the room without administering the medication. If this happens, return again in five minutes and state, "Jeff, it is time for your medicine now." Offer the child a choice, but not the choice of whether or not to take the medicine. He can choose a chaser for oral medications; or, within limits, the site for an injection; or he may want to swab the site with alcohol before the injection.

Most liquid medicines are flavored to make them more palatable. If the taste is objectionable, however, mix it with a small amount of syrup or honey. Never mix medicines with nutritional foods because the child may associate the bitter taste with the food and refuse the food later. Do not mix medications with a glass of liquid (even a medicine cupful may be too much) or a jar of baby food because the child will have to injest the entire amount to get his medication.

Pills may be crushed and mixed with honey if necessary. Enteric coated tablets and capsules are designed to dissolve in the intestines and must not be crushed before administering.

After administering medications (oral, ear drops, nose drops, or parenteral injections), stay with the child and comfort him as necessary. If he can have fluids, offer a drink of his choice, even if the medication was not an oral one; most children drink a great deal of liquid and will accept them at this time. This increases the child's intake and gives you an opportunity to comfort him. Visit him at other than medication times so that he does not associate you only with painful, restrictive, or intrusive procedures.

After an injection, the child (especially the preschooler) may want a bandage placed over the puncture site. Recall that the preschooler is concerned with bodily mutilation. He may think he will bleed through the injection site; the bandage restores his body integrity. Always record the injection site.

Oral Medications

In Figure 7-3 a dropper is used to give oral medications to the infant. Hold him securely in the cradle position as shown, and stabilize his head by pressing it to your body. Note that the infant's left arm is secured with nurse's left hand; his right arm is pressed between nurse's left arm and side (not shown). Reverse this hold if you are left-handed. If the dropper is to enter child's mouth, attach a short

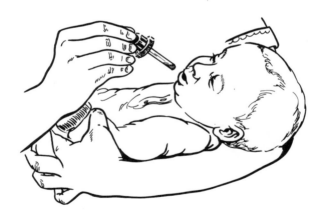

Figure 7-3.

length of tubing to dropper and place it to the back and side of child's mouth. Squeeze gently, allowing the child adequate time to swallow the medication. If no tubing is attached to dropper, do not place it in the child's mouth. Gently press on the infant's chin to open his mouth; then squirt a small amount of medication to the side and back of his mouth.

Figure 7-4 shows a nipple being used to give oral medications to the infant. If the taste is pleasant, the infant will suck. Hold the infant in cradle position and squirt (with a syringe with needle removed) or pour (from a medicine cup) medication into the nipple as the infant sucks. Follow medication with clear water, formula, or juice unless contraindicated.

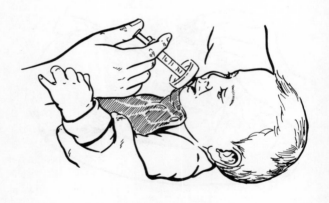

Figure 7-4.

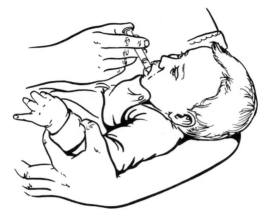

Figure 7-5.

In Figure 7-5 a syringe with the needle removed is used to offer oral medications. Hold the infant in cradle position and place the syringe to back and side of his mouth. Gently expel medication, allowing him time to swallow. The young child may enjoy getting his medication this way, via a "squirt," provided you show him first that the needle has been removed.

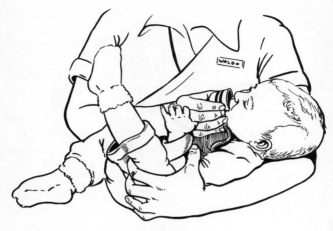

Figure 7-6.

Figure 7-6 illustrates oral medicines given from a cup. You must administer them slowly, allowing the child to swallow between sips. For the toddler and older child, simply hand them the cup.

Intramuscular Injections

Recommended injection sites for children are:

Ventrogluteal area (any age);
Vastus lateralis (infant and young child);
Rectus femoris (alternate site) for infant and young child;
Gluteal region (children who have been walking for at least one year);
Deltoid (any age).

Needle length and gauge *usually* used in children vary from a 25-gauge, 5/8-inch needle to a 22-gauge, one-inch-needle. Size and gauge will vary and should be selected for each child on an individual basis. The adolescent may require a 22-gauge, 1 1/2-inch needle for injections in the gluteus maximus.

Ventrogluteal (Hochstetter's) site

The muscles injected at the ventrogluteal site are the gluteus medius and minimus (Figure 7-7). This muscle mass is sufficiently thick, even in emaciated persons, and the subcutaneous tissue is less dense than over the gluteus maximus. This site contains

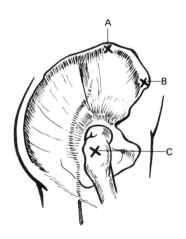

Figure 7-7.

no major nerves or vessels and a too-deep injection will reach only bone.

The site is easily located in a triangle within three palpable bony landmarks: iliac crest (A), anterior superior iliac spine (B), and the greater trochanter of the femur (C). In children, it often is not necessary to palpate the trochanter; the injection may be given directly below the iliac crest, in line with the lateral thigh. A distinct advantage of using the ventrogluteal site for injections in children is that it is accessible from practically any position (see following figures).

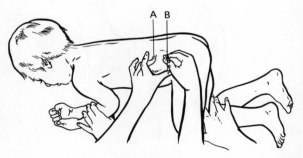

Figure 7-8.

Child turned on his side; assistant helps child to hold still by securing his arms and legs with her hands (Figure 7-8). Locate iliac crest (A) and anterior superior iliac spine (B), and give injection directly below iliac crest. Angle needle *slightly* toward crest.

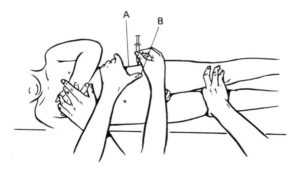

Figure 7-9.

Child lying in supine position near edge of bed (Figure 7-9). Assistant helps him to hold still by securing his hands on his chest and holding his legs right above the knees. Lean over child and locate iliac crest (A), and anterior superior iliac spine (B). (Note: in this drawing, the nurse has already moved her index finger from iliac crest to view the injection site.) Holding syringe parallel to bed, angle needle slightly toward iliac crest.

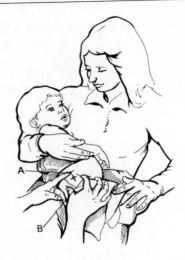

Figure 7-10.

Infant held in cradle position with arms and legs secured by mother or assistant (Figure 7-10). Palpate iliac crest (A) and anterior superior iliac spine (B). (Nurse's thumb is resting on gluteal muscle.) "X" denotes correct site. The ventrogluteal site can also be used with the infant held upright on an adult's shoulder as if for burping.

Vastus Lateralis and Rectus Femoris Sites

The muscles injected in the thigh are the vastus lateralis and the rectus femoris, two of the four muscles that comprise the quadriceps femoris muscle (Figure 7-11). Locate greater trochanter of femur and knee, then divide this area into thirds. Give injection in middle third, stabilizing thigh, and compressing slightly, as shown. For vastus lateralis (A), inject lateral thigh anterior to femur as shown (B); needle is perpendicular to thigh or slightly angled toward anterior thigh.

This muscle may also be injected by using an anterior approach lateral to the middle of the anterior thigh and directing the needle on a straight front-to-back course (as in (D) but more lateral).

To inject the rectus femoris muscle (C), angle needle on a straight front-to-back course in the midanterior portion of thigh as shown (D).

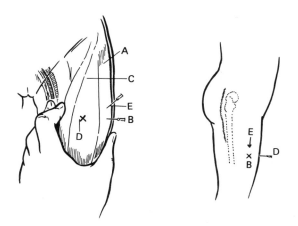

Figure 7-11.

An alternate approach to injections in the thigh is to inject the upper outer quadrant of the thigh with the needle directed at a 45-degree angle to the knee (E).

Posteriolateral Gluteal Site

The muscle most often used as an injection site in the posteriolateral gluteal region is the gluteus maximus. The gluteal region in infants is small and is composed primarily of fat; the musculature itself is poorly developed until the child has been walking for a year or more. For this reason, injections in this area may be dangerously close to the sciatic nerve. Johnson and Raptow state that the gluteal area is satisfactory for intramuscular injections *provided:* that the child is in the prone position; that the injection is given *perpendicular to the surface on which the child is lying* rather than perpendicular to the skin; and that the site is above a line connecting the posterior superior iliac spine and the greater trochanter of the femur. Because of the difficulty in properly positioning many infants and small children, this site is generally not recommended for the child under two years of age.

With child in prone position, locate posterior superior iliac spine (A) and greater trochanter of femur (B) (Figure 7-12). Draw an imaginary line connecting these two landmarks. The proper injection site ("X") will be above this line. Direct needle at a 90-degree angle to surface on which child is lying, *not* a 90-degree angle to the skin.

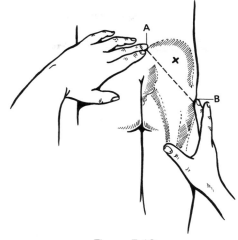

Figure 7-12.

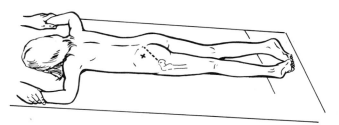

Figure 7-13.

Figure 7-13 shows the child in correct position for intramuscular injection in posteriolateral gluteal region. A "toe-in" position is used to relax the muscles.

Deltoid Site

The deltoid muscle is small in infants and young children (Figure 7-14); it can therefore accommodate only a small amount of medication. Thick, viscid medications should not be given in this site; in addition, repeated injections into the deltoid are painful.

The site ("X") is located between the acromion (A) and the armpit (B). For small children, measure one fingerbreadth below the acromion; for adolescents, measure three fingerbreadths. Grasp muscle at injection site and compress between thumb and fingers. Insert needle slightly upward toward shoulder.

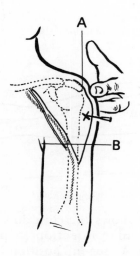

Figure 7-14.

Intravenous Medications

The most complex aspect of drug administration is the use of IV fluids as a vehicle for the administration of medications. Most advances in IV-drug administration, such as the minibottle, are used in adult nursing and are not generally appropriate for widespread use in the pediatric patient. Pediatric nurses must use such devices as the volume control chamber to dilute and deliver IV medications. The nurse must make decisions concerning the proper dilution, rate of administration, and possibility of incompatibility with other drugs. Table 7-1 offers guidelines for the administration of IV antibiotics.

Intravenous Retrograde Drug Administration

The retrograde method of administering intravenous medications permits a controlled concentration of a drug to be given over a controlled-time interval. This method eliminates the administration of a bolus of IV medication even if more than one drug must be given at the same time. It also permits the administration of drugs that are incompatible with the IV solution itself.

Equipment

Extension tubing with capacity to accommodate required volume of diluted drugs. For example: 4 ml volume: Venotube 20 inch (No. 4429 by Abbott); 50 ml volume: blood warming coil (No. 4663 by Abbott); 70 ml volume: blood warming coil (No. V5420 by McGaw). Tubing sizes will vary with the manufacturer. Do not use extension tubing with arms because air may become trapped in the arms.

Two 3-way stopcocks

Two stopcock plugs

Disposable syringes

Plain D₅W if IV solution is incompatible with drugs to be administered

Procedure

Select appropriate-size extension tubing. A 4-milliliter Venotube is usually adequate for the neonate; an infant may require two four-milliliter Venotubes; the older child may need a 50- or 70-milliliter (blood-warming coil) tubing volume. If the volume of diluted drug exceeds 70 milliliters, it may be divided and given successively over more than one hour.

Connect extension tubing and stopcocks between regular IV (including infusion controller/pump and filter) and the child (see Figure 7-16). Plug stopcocks with sterile plugs. Change extension tubing and stopcocks daily when regular IV tubing is changed.

Measure and draw up medication into syringe #1 (Figure 7-15), following manufacturer's directions for reconstitution. In syringe #2, draw up amount of diluent necessary for the desired concentration (see Table 7-1 or your institution's guidelines). Use child's IV solution for diluent if the drug is compatible with it. Use D₅W for diluent if IV solution is incompatible with drug; if heparin

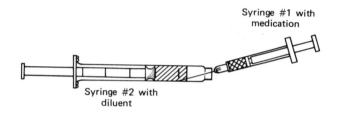

Syringe #1 with
medication

Syringe #2 with
diluent

Figure 7-15.

has been added to IV solution; if more than one
drug must be given at one time; or if IV solution is a
peripheral hyperalimentation fluid. (See Glucose
Barriers, below.)

To add reconstituted medication from syringe
#1 to diluent in syringe #2: remove needle from
syringe #2 and pull plunger back far enough to accommodate the medication; then add medication
through hub into syringe #2. Replace needle. Mix
drug and diluent by tipping syringe back and forth,
allowing air bubble to move from one end to the
other. Force air out of syringe.

Draw plunger back and forth on empty syringe
#3 to prevent it from sticking (Figure 7-16). Re-
move plug from stopcock (A) and needle from
syringe #3. Place plug in needle of syringe to maintain its sterility. Attach syringe to stopcock, being

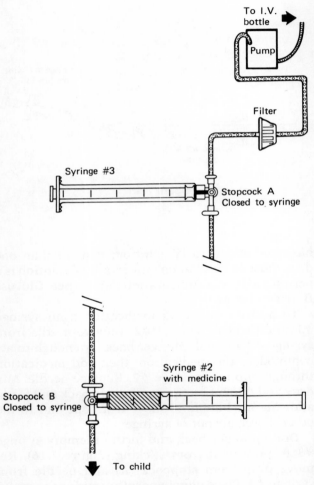

To I.V. bottle

Pump

Filter

Syringe #3

Stopcock A
Closed to syringe

Stopcock B
Closed to syringe

Syringe #2
with medicine

To child

Figure 7-16.

sure syringe is large enough to accommodate displaced IV solution.

Remove plug from stopcock (B) and needle from syringe #2. Place plug in needle. Attach syringe #2 with diluted medication to stopcock. Hold syringe perpendicular to stopcock and aspirate air bubble from stopcock (bubble will rise and stay in top of syringe).

Turn stopcock (B) *off* to child and stopcock (A) *off* to IV line (Figure 7 - 17). If an IV controller or pump is used, turn it off unless the flow rate is less than 10 ml/hour.

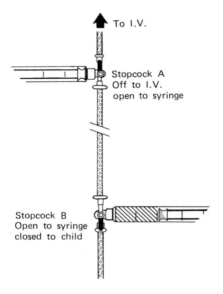

To I.V.

Stopcock A
Off to I.V.
open to syringe

Stopcock B
Open to syringe
closed to child

Figure 7-17.

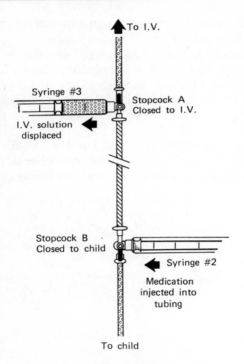

To I.V.

Syringe #3

Stopcock A
Closed to I.V.

I.V. solution
displaced

Stopcock B
Closed to child

Syringe #2

Medication
injected into
tubing

To child

Figure 7-18.

Inject medication (syringe #2) retrograde into
extension tubing (Figure 7-18). IV solution will be
displaced into syringe #3 as medication fills the
extension tubing; this solution is discarded. Turn
stopcock (A), then (B), back to open IV line. Remove
syringes, replace stopcock plugs, and check all connections to be sure they are tight. Record medication on flowsheet.

Glucose Barriers
Glucose barriers are necessary when the medication and IV solution are incompatible or when more than one drug must be given at the same time. Use the following guidelines for glucose barriers:

Flow Rate	Amount of Glucose
Less than 10 ml/hr	1 ml
10 to 20 ml/hr	2 to 3 ml
20 to 50 ml/hr	3 to 5 ml

When administering two drugs, draw up necessary amount of glucose barrier and inject retrograde between the two drugs to prevent their admixture. If the drug and IV solution are incompatible, use two glucose barriers, injecting one before and one after the medication. When changing syringes, turn stopcock (B) one-eighth turn so that it is closed to all three parts.

Volume Control Chamber Medications
If your institution does not use the retrograde method of administering IV medications, drugs may be added to the IV solution via the volume control chamber (Figure 6-16). However, care must be taken to assure that the IV does not contain heparin or additives other than glucose and electrolytes. Only one drug may be given at a time using this method.

Another disadvantage of this method is that the volume chamber frequently contains more fluid than is necessary for the administration of the medication. For example: the medication is mixed in 10 milliliters, and the volume chamber has been filled to 40 milliliters. The flow rate is 20 milliliters per hour. If you add the 10 milliliters of medication to the volume chamber, you have a total of 50 milliliters, which will take two and one-half hours to empty at a flow rate of 20 ml/hr. It may then be necessary to invert the control chamber and IV bottle and to squeeze the chamber to return a portion of fluid to the bottle before adding the medication. Be sure to subtract the amount returned from the IV flow record. This policy varies with institutions.

Ear Drops

To instill ear drops place the child in mummy restraint if necessary and turn his head to unaffected

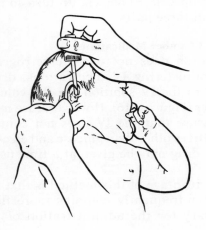

Figure 7-19.

side (Figure 7-19). For the child under three years of age, hold pinna of ear down and back as shown; for older children and adults, hold pinna up and back. Drop *warm* ear drops in external canal; keep child in this position for a few minutes to allow drops to run onto eardrum.

Nose Drops

Hold the infant in cradle position when administering nose drops. Tilt his head back and stabilize it in the crook of your arm by pressing it between your arm and body (Figure 7-20). Squeeze drops into each nostril as prescribed. Place the older child supine on a bed with a pillow under his shoulders so that his head hyperextends over the pillow. Ask him to sniff after you instill the drops.

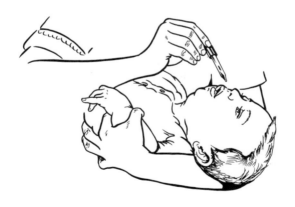

Figure 7-20.

Table 7-1. Parameters for Commonly Administered
Intravenous Antibiotics in Pediatrics

Antibiotics	Recommended Pediatric Dosage Ranges	May be Given IV Push?
Amikacin (Amikin)	*Newborns:* 10 mg/kg initially, followed by 15 mg/kg/24 hr Divided into 2 doses *Older Infants and Children:* 15 mg/kg/24 hr Divided into 2–3 doses	NO
Ampicillin	*Under* 40 kg: *Moderately severe infection:* 50–100 mg/kg/24 hr Divided into 4 doses *Severe infections:* 200 mg/kg/24 hr Divided into 4–6 doses *Moderately severe infections:* 1–2g/24 hr Divided into 4–6 doses *Severe infections:* Up to 8–14 g/24 hr Divided into 4–6 doses	Yes—use within 1 hr and administer slowly

May be Given via Metriset?	Minimum Dilution for IV Drip	Minimum Infusion Time	Commonly Encountered IV Incompatibilities
Yes	250 mg/100 ml	30–60 min/ dose; infants should receive 1–2 hr infusion	SHOULD NOT BE MIXED WITH ANY OTHER DRUGS IN IV FLUID
Yes—use within 1 hr	1 g/10 ml	200 mg/min	SHOULD NOT BE MIXED WITH ANY OTHER DRUGS IN IV FLUID

Table 7-1. (continued)

Antibiotics	Recommended Pediatric Dosage Ranges	May be Given IV Push?
Carbenicillin (Geopen, Pyopen)	*Urinary tract infections (Pseudomonas):* 50–200 mg/kg/24 hr Divided into 6 doses *Severe urinary tract and other infections (Pseudomonas):* 400–500 mg/kg/24 hr Divided into 6 doses *Urinary tract infections (Proteus and E. Coli):* 50–100 mg/kg/24 hr Divided into 4–6 doses *Severe urinary tract and other infections (Proteus and E. Coli):* 300–400/kg/24 hr Divided into 4–6 doses	Yes—Dilute 1 g in no less than 5 ml; administer slowly
Cefazolin (Kefzol, Ancef)	*Moderate infections:* 25–50mg/kg/24 hr Divided into 3–4 doses *Severe infections:* 100 mg/kg/24 hr Divided into 3–4 doses Not recommended for premature infants or infants less than 1 month of age	Yes—Dilute 1 g in no less than 10ml; administer over 3–5 min

May be Given via Metriset?	Minimum Dilution for IV Drip	Minimum Infusion Time	Commonly Encountered IV Incompatibilities
Yes	1 g/10 ml	15 min/dose	Isuprel Tetracyclines Chloramphenicol Gentamicin
Yes	1 g/50 ml	15–30 min/dose	SHOULD NOT BE MIXED WITH ANY OTHER DRUGS IN IV FLUID

Table 7-1. **(continued)**

Antibiotics	Recommended Pediatric Dosage Ranges	May be Given IV Push?
Cephalothin (Keflin)	*Most susceptible infections:* 50 mg/kg/24 hr Divided into 4 doses *Severe infections:* 100 mg/kg/24 hr Divided into 4 doses *Life-threatening infections and lowered resistance:* 80–225 mg/kg/24 hr Maximum of 12 g Divided into 4–6 doses	Yes—In a concentration of up to 100 mg/ml; administer over 3–5 min
Chloramphenicol (Chloromycetin)	*Premature and full-term infants (up to 2 weeks):* 25 mg/kg/24 hr Divided into 4 doses *Infants over 2 weeks and older children:* 50 mg/kg/24 hr Divided into 4 doses *Severe infections:* 100 mg/kg/24 hr Divided into 4 doses	Yes—Dilute 1 g in no less than 10 ml; administer over at least 1 min
Clindamycin (Cleocin)	*Moderately severe infections:* 15–25 mg/kg/24 hr Divided into 3–4 doses *Severe infections:* 25–40 mg/kg/24 hr Divided into 3–4 doses Not recommended for infants less than 1 month of age	No

May be Given via Metriset?	Minimum Dilution for IV Drip	Minimum Infusion Time	Commonly Encountered IV Incompatibilities
Yes	1 g/10 ml	200 mg/min	Aminophylline Hydrocortisone phosphate Aqua-Mephyton Sodium bicarbonate Tetracyclines Chloramphenicol Gentamicin Oxacillin
Yes	In any convenienct amount	**	Ampicillin Aminophylline Digoxin Solu-Cortef Solu-Medrol Aqua-Mephyton Carbenicillin Keflin Tetracyclines Vitamin B complex with C Oxacillin
Yes	300 mg/50 ml	30 mg/min	Solu-Cortef Vitamin B complex with C Ampicillin Aminophylline

Table 7-1. **(continued)**

Antibiotics	Recommended Pediatric Dosage Ranges	May be Given IV Push?
Erythromycin Glucoheptonate	*Moderately severe infections:* 40–50 mg/kg/24 hr Divided into 4 doses *Severe infections:* 60–70 mg/kg/24 hr Divided into 4 doses	No
Erythromycin Lactobionate	15–20 mg/kg/24 hr Divided into 4 doses	Yes—In a concentration of 10 mg/ml; administer slowly
Gentamicin (Garamycin)	*Infants and neonates:* 6 mg/kg/24 hr Divided into 2 doses *Less than 2 years of age:* 2–3 mg/kg/24 hr Divided into 2–3 doses *Over 20 kg:* *Urinary tract infections:* 0.8–1.2 mg/kg/24 hr Divided into 3 doses *Other infections:* 3–5 mg/kg/24 hr Divided into 3 doses	No
Kanamycin (Kantrex)	*Less than 7 days of age:* 15–20 mg/kg/24 hr Divided into 2 doses *Greater than 7 days of age:* 20–30 mg/kg/24 hr Divided into 2–3 doses	No

May be Given via Metriset?	Minimum Dilution for IV Drip	Minimum Infusion Time	Commonly Encountered IV Incompatibilities
Yes	500 mg/100 ml	20–60 min/dose	Aminophylline Heparin sodium Solu-Cortef Vitamin B complex with C
Yes	500 mg/100 ml	20 min/dose	SHOULD NOT BE MIXED WITH ANY OTHER DRUGS IN IV FLUID
Yes	1 mg/ml	30–60 min/dose	SHOULD NOT BE MIXED WITH ANY OTHER DRUGS IN IV FLUID
Yes	25 mg/10 ml	7.5 mg/min	SHOULD NOT BE MIXED WITH ANY OTHER DRUGS IN IV FLUID

Table 7-1. (continued)

Antibiotics	Recommended Pediatric Dosage Ranges	May be Given IV Push?
Lincomycin (Lincocin)	10–20 mg/kg/24 hr Divided into 2–3 doses Not recommended for infants less than 1 month of age	No
Methicillin (Staphcillin)	100 mg/kg/24 hr Divided into 4–6 doses	Yes—But only in emergency. Dilute 100 mg in no less than 5 ml; administer 10 ml/min
Minocycline (Minocin)	4 mg/kg initially followed by 4 mg/kg/24 hr Divided into 2 doses	No
Nafcillin (Unipen)	*Newborns:* 20 mg/kg/24 hr Divided into 2 doses *Older infants and children:* 50 mg/kg/24 hr Divided into 2 doses May double dose in severe infections	Yes—But only cautiously

May be Given via Metriset?	Minimum Dilution for IV Drip	Minimum Infusion Time	Commonly Encountered IV Incompatibilities
Yes	1 g/100 ml	15 mg/min	Kanamycin Carbenicillin Cloxacillin
Yes	1 g/50 ml	200 mg/min	SHOULD NOT BE MIXED WITH ANY OTHER DRUGS IN IV FLUID
Yes	10 mg/100 ml	60 min/dose	SHOULD NOT BE MIXED WITH ANY OTHER DRUGS IN IV FLUID
Yes	1 g/30 ml	200 mg/min	SHOULD NOT BE MIXED WITH ANY OTHER DRUGS IN IV FLUID

Table 7-1. (continued)

Antibiotics	Recommended Pediatric Dosage Ranges	May be Given IV Push?
Oxacillin (Prostaphlin)	*Neonates and premature infants:* 25 mg/kg/24 hr Divided into 4–6 doses *Under 40 kg:* 50–100 mg/kg/24 hr Divided into 4–6 doses *Over 40 kg:* 1–6 g/24 hr Divided into 4–6 doses	Yes—Dilute 1 g in at least 10 ml; administer over 10 min
Penicillin G Potassium	*Premature and full-term newborns:* 60,000 units/kg/24 hr Divided into 2 doses *Older children:* 25,000–50,000 units/ kg/24 hr Divided into 4–6 doses *Severe infections* (meningitis): 300,000–400,000 units/kg/24 hr Divided into 4–6 doses	Not recommended

May be Given via Metriset?	Minimum Dilution for IV Drip	Minimum Infusion Time	Commonly Encountered IV Incompatibilities
Yes	1 g/10 ml	100 mg/min	Keflin K Penicillin G Tetracyclines Chloramphenicol Aqua-Mephyton
Yes	In any con-venient amount*	**	SHOULD NOT BE MIXED WITH ANY OTHER DRUGS IN IV FLUID

Table 7-1. (continued)

Antibiotics	Recommended Pediatric Dosage Ranges	May be Given IV Push?
Tetracycline	*Newborn—not recommended:* 10–15 mg/kg/24 hr Divided into 2 doses *Older infants and children:* 10–20 mg/kg/24 hr Divided into 2 doses	Yes—Do not exceed a rate of 10 mg/min
Tobramycin (Nebcin)	*Neonates:* Up to 4 mg/kg/24 hr Divided into 2 doses *Children and older infants:* Serious infections: 3 mg/kg/24 hr Divided into 3 doses Life-threatening infections: 5 mg/kg/24 hr Divided into 3–4 doses	No

May be Given via Metriset?	Minimum Dilution for IV Drip	Minimum Infusion Time	Commonly Encountered IV Incompatibilities
Yes	10 mg/ml	20 mg/min	Aminophylline Lasix Heparin Sodium Solu-Cortef Vitamin B complex with C Ampicillin Keflin Chloramphenicol K Penicillin G Nafcillin Methicillin Sodium bicarbonate Solu-Medrol Oxacillin
Yes	25–50 ml	20–60 min/ dose	SHOULD NOT BE MIXED WITH ANY OTHER DRUGS IN IV FLUID

Table 7-1. (continued)

Antibiotics	Recommended Pediatric Dosage Ranges	May be Given IV Push?
Vancomycin (Vancocin)	44 mg/kg/24 hr Divided into 4 doses	No

May be Given via Metriset?	Minimum Dilution for IV Drip	Minimum Infusion Time	Commonly Encountered IV Incompatibilities
Yes	500 mg/100 ml	25 mg/min	Chloramphenicol Tetracyclines Heparin sodium Methicillin K Penicillin G Aqua-Mephyton Sodium bicarbonate Vitamin B complex with C

*Manufacturer states that infusion time does not affect blood levels in the body. For the patients' safety, however, a given dose should be infused over no less than one-minute period. Infusion should also be completed within six hours.
**Information not available from manufacturer.

BIBLIOGRAPHY

Benzing, G. B. and Loggie, J. A New Retrograde Method For Administering Drugs Intravenously. *Pediatrics* 52:420, 1973.

Brandt, P. A., Smith, M. E., Ashburn, S. S., Graves, J. IM Injections in Children. *American Journal of Nursing* 72:1402, 1972.

Johnson, E. W. and Raptow, A.D. A Study of Intragluteal Injections. *Archives of Physical Medicine and Rehabilitation* 46:167–177, 1965.

Metheny, N. M. and Snively, W. D. *Nurse's Handbook of Fluid Balance* Ed. 2. Philadelphia, J. B. Lippincott Co., 1974, p. 292.

Robinson, L. A. and Whitacre, N. F. Intravenous Administration of Antibiotics in Children. *Pediatric Nursing* 3:21, 1977.

DATE DUE
